THE TOXIN TERMINATOR

Finding Focus, Energy and Renewed Health by Removing Hidden Toxins

By

Aimee Carlson

Dedication

My son Nicholas, my husband Curtis, my brother Jim and my father Gordon, who without their loving presence in my life I would not be the woman, wife, mother and grandmother that I am today.

Nicholas, you will never know just how God knew exactly what he was doing when he sent you to be my son. Because of you I am here today, able to share my experience, strength and hope with others who still suffer. Knowing I had the responsibility to be your mom brought me out of some of the darkest places in our lives. I am forever grateful for the gift of having you as my son!

My late brother Jim, who is my hero. He taught me what it looks like to live selflessly and through his death, he showed me how great my faith truly is.

My husband, Curt, you are my best friend, confidant and partner in this incredible journey called life. Your unwavering support gives me the strength to do the scary things, to walk into the unknown and to always be stepping forward!

And lastly, to my father Gordon. You have been my rock from the time I can remember. You taught me to never settle, you pushed me to want better, to be better to always challenge myself. I learned how to be the best businessperson I could be, from watching and learning from you.

Acknowledgements

The Environmental Working Group

The Centers for Disease Control and Prevention

PubMed

The American Cancer Society

The Environmental Protection Agency

The Federal Food and Drug Administration

Safer Cosmetics

Special Thanks

Thank you to Christie Ruffino, Laura Petersen and Alison Melody who encouraged me to bring this book to life. I also want to thank Travis Chappell, without your course the podcast would have never started and I wouldn't have met the most amazing people who have contributed to my journey in living a toxin free lifestyle. Thank you to the beautiful women who are so brave and vulnerable to share their stories; Libby Wright, Naomi Damask, Bobbi Schaben, Melissa Rupp, Sarah Steele and Donna EG Haugen. And lastly, thank you to Skyla Mann, my mentor and biggest cheerleader, believing in me long before I did.

Contents

Introduction

Learn the five pillars of living a toxin-free lifestyle, so that you can prevent chronic disease, reverse chronic disease and renew your focus, energy and live a long healthy life.

This book will walk you down the path of a toxin-free lifestyle and give you the tools to detox and cleanse your life and environment. It will also share the stories of so many who have struggled with their health, just like you and me!

I have had the privilege of learning from some of the best healers, doctors, practitioners and thought leaders in the natural field, as I have experienced my own renewed health over the past seven years. In hosting my own podcast, The Toxin Terminator, I have heard many inspirational stories of people overcoming chronic diseases, including cancer, autoimmune diseases, Crohn's Disease and Meniere's Disease, by removing toxins from their lifestyles to allow their bodies to fully heal. I have completely immersed myself into this toxin- free lifestyle to bring my teachings to those who still suffer.

This book will look at the current state of health our nation is in, how our bodies have the natural ability to heal itself, and what toxic overload may look like. You'll learn how to pay attention to the signals your body is giving you, whether it is gently nudging you with a whisper or screaming at you waving the white flag! As the chapters unfold you will discover the five pillars to living a toxin-free lifestyle with each pillar bringing you the toxins to avoid as well as the safe alternatives you can use to renew your health. There are many toxins we are exposed to on a daily basis; through our homes, work and the environment. This book will focus on the toxins we are exposed to within our homes and more importantly the ones we are exposed to on a daily basis. By focusing on these, we can take the steps to have a greater impact on our overall health.

Kristi Cronin, Nurse Practioner and Author~

"As a health care provider this podcast has challenged me to continue to think about my patients as a whole. I am typically one of the more conservative providers when it comes to prescribing medications and these discussions continue to support my belief to put the

 patient first and consider all appropriate forms of treatment, including alternative forms."

Dr. Al Lundeen, Chiropractor, Life Coach and host of RiseUp!Radio show~

"All the episodes have left me with applicable ideas of how to create a healthier environment for my kids and for myself. Amazing podcast!"

Dr. Kyrin Dunstan, Podcast host of Her Brilliant Health Revolution~

"Vital topic and fantastic presentation for the details of how you can protect yourself, while living in this toxic soup that we all live in. Doctors are not teaching this, so it's essential to get this info and thank you, Aimee for sharing with us!"

Dr. Tabatha Barber, Author, Podcast Host of The Functional Gynecologist Podcast~

"Aimee has done an awesome job at bringing this important information to light! As a physician, I'm so happy to see people talking about our environmental toxins and how they impact our health. So, thank you!!"

My Story

I have been an entrepreneur my entire adult life. I grew up in my family's business, an automotive franchise, where we performed preventative vehicle maintenance. I learned the business from the bottom up, starting as a cashier, then learning to work on the cars and becoming ASE Certified through our training. When my father decided we needed a family member in Des Moines to fill a management position, as well as have eyes in the market there, I was asked to fulfill that need. I learned how to become a manager, eventually becoming a district manager and finally owning the business. Not only was I exposed to environmental toxins on a daily basis as I worked on the vehicles, but the entrepreneurial mindset of owning your business can be quite toxic to our emotions. I was always looking to improve our services, better the customer experience, improve the bottom line and offer the highest quality of work experience to our employees. As the owner, it wasn't just me and my family's well-being on the line. The decisions I made, were also affecting my 50 employees and their families. Owning and operating your business creates a lot of stress on the body and requires many sacrifices. For many years, I worked 60-70 hours a week. It wasn't until my son was seven years old, that we were able to take our first vacation. Many plans were made but had to be cancelled. When you own the business, and things go wrong, you have to step in and get things going. Working in the fast-paced environment of a quick lube, the food choices you make are never the best. Sometimes I didn't eat all day or crammed in fast food, when the time allowed. The never being good enough mentality, the stress of owning your own business and the daily exposures of chemicals at work and at home, the poor diet choices and lack of any type of exercise, began to take a toll on my overall health.

In the beginning, I had weird unexplainable symptoms. One time, I had an abscess on my face. I woke up one morning with the left side of my face so swollen, that I had no jawline. I ended up having to have tubes put in to drain it and plastic surgery to avoid scarring. Another time I had canker sores in my mouth and throat so bad (I think they said over 50) that they had to numb my mouth, so I could eat. I developed allergies that I never had before and was put on medications. I suffered from headaches almost daily. Eventually I began having migraines that would cause me to lose my vision on the left side. I was also nauseated and extremely light sensitive with those migraines. At the age of 37, after working with doctors for years on my cycle issues, I had a partial hysterectomy because no medications were helping. It had already been determined prior to my surgery, that I was in perimenopause. The average woman starts menopause at the age of 47-51. After my hysterectomy, the surgeon said that they found pre-cancerous cells in my uterus. He said that it was a good thing it had been removed. I struggled with my emotions for years, feeling like I was on a constant roller coaster. I was either really happy and energetic or melancholy and numb. There really weren't any in between. I didn't sleep well and had a hard time focusing. At the time, I blamed this on menopause. At one point, my husband thought I should be tested for being bipolar.

During this time, I was no longer working daily in the stores. I really did not consider myself to be unhealthy. I ran and worked out and certainly wasn't overweight. I truly thought that many of the issues I had were just stress and normal aging processes. At least, that is what the doctors told me. Not once did any of the doctors provide me with any tools to handle the stress in my life. In fact, I was put on antidepressants and hormones. Even writing this now, I can see that I had no idea how bad I felt. I think when you have symptoms that gradually keep piling on, you become acclimated to them. That's not to say you like them. It's just that you don't know there is any different way to feel. I had decided this was just how life was going to be. It wasn't until I went to a class hosted by my friend, that I started my journey into learning about my health. She had been inviting me to one of "those" classes for over a year. I knew it was one of those salesy pyramid things and I had zero interest in going. After a year of invites, I finally gave in and went. I truly just wanted to get her to stop bugging me!! It was a class on essential oils. Before you say anything, let me say that I was the biggest skeptic ever. I thought essential oils were for hippies and using them meant you didn't bathe and sat around a campfire singing Kumbaya! As the oils were passed around, I really thought they stunk. I couldn't understand how anyone would want to use them. The only one I liked was peppermint. Boy, I couldn't get enough of it. I listened to the stories that were shared and what they said these essential oils could do. I honestly didn't believe it. It was probably because I really had zero exposure to any kind of alternative medicine. I knew that medicines weren't working for me, so how were these bottles of oils going to really help? After the class was over, I asked my friend if she had anything in her bag of tricks that would help me sleep and not wake up in a pile of sweat. She offered me something and I tried it. I thought what can it hurt, right? I actually slept for the first time through the night and was not drenched. I had no idea what it was, but I couldn't get my hands on it fast enough. This experience led me down a path of learning about alternative ways to heal our bodies. More importantly, I learned about toxins, where they are, what they do to our bodies and how I could limit my exposure to them within the four walls of our home. I learned that many of the products I was using every day, were loaded with ingredients that were poisoning my body and contributing to my chronic disease. As I slowly began to remove toxins, I began to feel better. I was allowing my body to do what it naturally wants to do, heal. I just had to give it the chance, by detoxing and cleansing. Removing what I cleaned our home with and what I did laundry with, were some of the first things I changed. I'm happy to report that I haven't had a migraine since then. It took me over two years to remove most of the toxins in my home, and I'm learning more every single day. I don't think the journey will ever end, since new information comes out all the time. As we peel the layers, we get to find new things to optimize our health. I truly believe that is what we need to do. In my case, it wasn't possible to detox everything at once. I think that was also God's plan for me. I had to learn these pillars one by one and implement them as I learned. What I do know, is that at 54, I have better sleep, better focus, more energy and mentally I am the best version of me I have ever been!! I am truly living the best part of my life and feel better now than I did in my 30's.

Removing toxins has had such a profound effect on me, that I started sharing what I was experiencing with my family and friends. Before I knew it, I had a team of over 200 people in my network marketing company. The idea that that one meeting changed my life and I could turn around and change others was surreal to me. When I am teaching others and helping them get healthy, I am in my happy place. About a year ago, I started a podcast, The Toxin Terminator. I wanted to be able to share stories of people like me, who were overcoming chronic disease by removing toxins. I have interviewed many guests, who have shared their stories, their expertise and their modalities to help us all live a toxin-free lifestyle. I believe that I have truly stepped into God's purpose for me. It is to help others remove hidden toxins and find hope. My desire for you is that you read something on the following pages that gently nudges you, or perhaps you are like me and it slaps you upside the head. It will get you started in taking those first steps to a toxin-free lifestyle!

Chapter One: What is Chronic Disease?

According to the (Centers for Disease Control and Prevention, n.d.) six in ten Americans live with at least one chronic disease. Chronic diseases are the leading cause of death and disability in the United States and are also the leading driver of health care costs. As a nation, we spend over $3.3 trillion dollars each year on health care and that number continues to rise each year!

Chronic disease is defined as a disease or illness lasting one year or more requiring medical attention or limits daily activities, or both. Some examples of chronic disease are heart disease, cancer and diabetes. The NCCDPHP acknowledges that toxic exposures, diet and exercise are leading behaviors for acquiring a chronic disease. That's great news for us!! It means just as we can contribute to chronic disease, we can prevent it too!! The American Cancer Society (American Cancer Society, n.d.) states that 42-45% of all cancer cases are preventable, by modifying our risk behaviors, such as how we move, what we eat and our environmental toxins.

Here's a more comprehensive list of chronic diseases found in Medline plus.gov (Medlineplus.gov, n.d.):

- Alzheimer's disease and dementia
- Arthritis
- Asthma
- Cancer
- COPD
- Crohn's disease
- Cystic fibrosis
- Diabetes
- Epilepsy
- Heart disease
- HIV/AIDS
- Mood disorders (bipolar, cyclothymic, and depression)
- Multiple sclerosis
- Parkinson's disease

Here's a great graphic that presents this information in a visual format that highlights all of the above data.

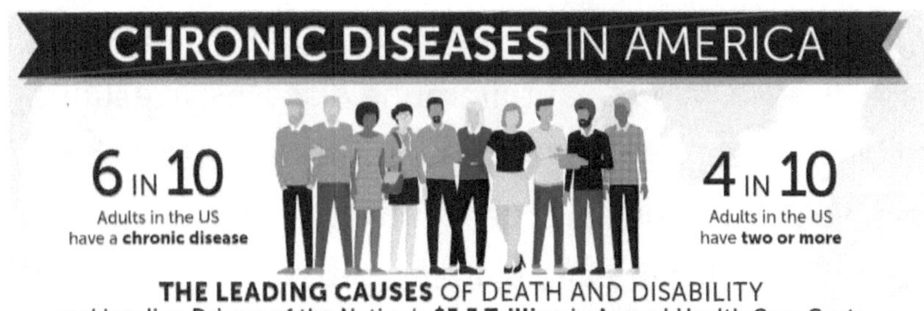

I believe that the rise of chronic disease in our society, is due to the increase of toxic exposures in our environments. We, as a society, are creating these synthetic toxic chemicals in the name of science, beauty, medicine and progress. You name it, and we're creating it. The agencies that are supposed to be protecting us are not. Unfortunately, as you can see by the statistics above, this is all coming at a price. It is a price on our overall health and on our environment. I don't know about you, but when I look around, I am seeing more and more women suffering from infertility issues. There are also more kids with allergies, autism, ADHD and focus issues. Our children are developing faster. (National Children's Study, n.d.) shows the effects that our environmental toxins are having on our children. Many of my friends, who are doctors, are reporting seeing girls as young as eight years old with their menstrual cycles. We are becoming numb to the word cancer, when just a few short years ago it was a rare disease. We see autoimmune diseases, like lupus, celiac disease, arthritis and multiple sclerosis on the rise. We also struggle at being able to balance our hormones. Obesity and diabetes are commonplace. In fact, from State of Childhood Obesity (Obesity Rates &

Trends Data, n.d.), childhood obesity increased from 10% in 1994 to 18.5% in 2016. For adults, that number went from 22.9% in 1994 to 42.4% in 2018. According to the CDC (Centers for Disease Control & Prevention) (Diabetes Data, n.d.), in 1958, there were only 1.58 million people in the United States with diabetes, while there are now over 34.2 million people with the disease. They go on to state that your risk of death is 60% higher, compared to someone who does not have diabetes. An even scarier statistic is that one out of five adults have no idea they have diabetes. Have you taken a look at your parents' medicine cabinet? Our elderly population is on more medications than they can keep track of. I hadn't even heard of the word dementia or Alzheimer's, when I was growing up. Now, we can't build memory care units fast enough to handle the demand. According to the CDC, (Mental Health, n.d.) today more than 50% of our population is suffering from a mental illness, and one in 25 Americans lives with a serious mental illness, such as schizophrenia, bipolar disorder, or major depression.

We have grown into a society that wants everything immediately, such as a great job, new house, fancy car and exotic vacation. The demands of these material things are creating stress on our bodies. We are keeping ourselves so busy, that we don't take the time to walk in nature or pick up a book. We are demanding many different convenience products, including packaged meals. We have more technology, which can be a good thing. However, it is removing the humanness of community. We all are spending more time on technology, instead of cultivating the relationships around us. That technology also has its own toxicity, especially Wi-Fi and the new 5G.

Do you agree with me that this is wrong? How do we get on top of it? What do we need to look at? First, we need to be informed. We need to learn just what is in our control, so that we can have an impact on these numbers. It's time to take our heads out of the sand. It's time to understand that you have to be your biggest advocate. I believe Big Pharma is making a lot of money from all of us that is truly keeping us sick! When is the last time your doctor asked you about your lifestyle? Did they sit down with you and let you know that the food choices you were making, were affecting your overall health? If you're like me, the answer is no. They just grab the prescription tablet. Look at the long list of side effects on any one of the commercials you see. Speaking of commercials, why is it necessary to have commercials about pharmaceutical drugs that can only be prescribed by a doctor? Do you think there is money behind them? Now don't get me wrong, I think there is absolutely a time and a place for doctors and medicine. I also believe there are many good doctors out there. Most of them, however, have been trained to treat a symptom. I believe the worlds of western medicine and holistic medicine should work together, as we look to get to the root of our symptoms. We shouldn't just put a band aid on them. The agencies that are supposed to be protecting you, simply are not. I used to think if it's sold in the store, then surely it must be safe. I didn't question it, because I didn't know better. According to the EPA (Environmental Protection Agency) (EPA, n.d.), there are over 86,000 chemicals in use today. However, there have been very few studies that have been done to test their safety for human consumption. The laws and regulations governing the safety of our products have gone largely unchanged since 1938. A new law, The Personal Care Products Safety Act, was introduced in the U.S. Congress in 2019, but as of the date of this writing, it has not yet been passed. In Europe, they have banned over 1300 chemicals for use in the beauty industry. In the United States, only eight chemicals have been banned. Yes, you heard that right. These are the facts in black and white. This lack of facts is why I am so passionate about sharing what these toxins are doing to us and where we can find them. In 2015, the EPA (EPA, n.d.) created a document called, Advancing Safer Chemicals in Products. This document shows that consumers are pushing to identify and remove hazardous chemicals. It is the beginning of the government and third parties working together to, at a minimum, provide information for consumers to make informed purchasing decisions. However, we still have a long way to go in mandating proper labeling and the use of non-toxic ingredients.

There are toxins everywhere. I don't want to scare you into believing that nothing is safe. This topic can get very overwhelming and frightening. We must focus on what we have control over, which is what happens inside the four walls of our homes. It's important to know the information on why we would even want to take a look at this. When I was first learning about toxins, I thought of chemical plants and MSDS sheets (material safety data sheets) that we had to use in our stores. I didn't associate toxins with the products that I was using every day in my home or my environment. Your environment includes the places you spend time in, from your home to your workplace to your car. It can include restaurants, movie theaters and stores, as well as nature. Your environment also consists of the people you associate with, the music you listen to, the television you watch and the books you read. For the purposes of this book, the focus will be within the four walls of your home. As I go through each pillar of living a toxin free lifestyle, I'll address the specific toxins, why they are considered a toxin and give you tools to make better choices. Every person is different, since we each have our own personal needs and lifestyles. Our body chemistry is also different. There are going to be parts that you don't relate to, that is OK. We get to take what we need and leave the rest.

Chapter Two: How does the Body Detox?

Our bodies are fearfully and wonderfully made. God designed our bodies to be able to nurture and heal ourselves naturally. We have a beautiful system to remove toxins. Our bodies natural detox system consists of the skin, lungs, blood, liver, kidneys and our lymphatic system. Each of these parts of this system play an integral role in removing toxins from our body. This is how we stay healthy and keep inflammation out of our bodies.

The skin is considered a sensory organ. It is the largest organ for protection and defense. It is responsible for temperature regulation, secretion and excretion. The skin plays an important role in the elimination of toxins and can assist the kidneys in their work. There have been studies which have detected heavy metals, phthalates and BPA's in our sweat. This shows that toxins can and are being released through our sweat (PubMed, n.d.).

Rashes can also be a symptom of detox. If there are too many toxins to be removed through our bowels or kidneys, we can have hives or rashes develop, as the skin attempts to push out what is irritating it. You can even experience breakouts, as the toxins are leaving the pores of your skin. While these can be bothersome, it actually is a good sign that your body is expelling the toxins. Sometimes they can be more than bothersome. If that happens, I tell people to slow down, use less of what you've been using, drink more water and take Epsom salt baths. I had horrible rashes on my armpits, when I switched to a natural deodorant. It didn't seem to matter what I tried. I developed the same rash. I then went to no deodorant at all, which worked pretty well. However, occasionally I would not like to be around myself. If you get my drift. I have finally found salt rock to work the best for me in the protection from odor. It still allows my body to sweat and does not release toxins or produce rashes.

After taking all the nutrients, minerals and enzymes that we need from our food, the excess is processed through our kidneys and livers and removed through urination. We also remove toxins through our bowel movements. When we are not eliminating from our bodies, the toxins build up and damage the enzymes. They displace the structural minerals causing damage to our bones, damage our internal organs and our DNA and interfere with our hormones. (Joseph Pizzorno, n.d.) We should be having bowel movements at least twice a day, preferably after each time you eat. When we don't, we are building up toxins, which are fermenting in our gut. This is what will produce bloating and gas for many of us. Have you heard of the Bristol stool chart? It shows us the types of stools we might have and helps us in identifying our stools. The frequency of our bowel movements is one of the easiest ways to know how healthy our digestive system is. I know it sounds funny. When I first started down this path, I had a mentor named Sonya Swan. Whenever anyone asked about a particular health issue, her first question was always, how's your poop? How we are eliminating from our bodies, is an easy way to know how healthy our gut is, as well as the rest of our body. In this chart below, we should be striving for Type 3 at least once or twice a day. When we don't eliminate the waste from our bodies, it builds up and ferments. This creates even more toxins.

Bristol Stool Chart

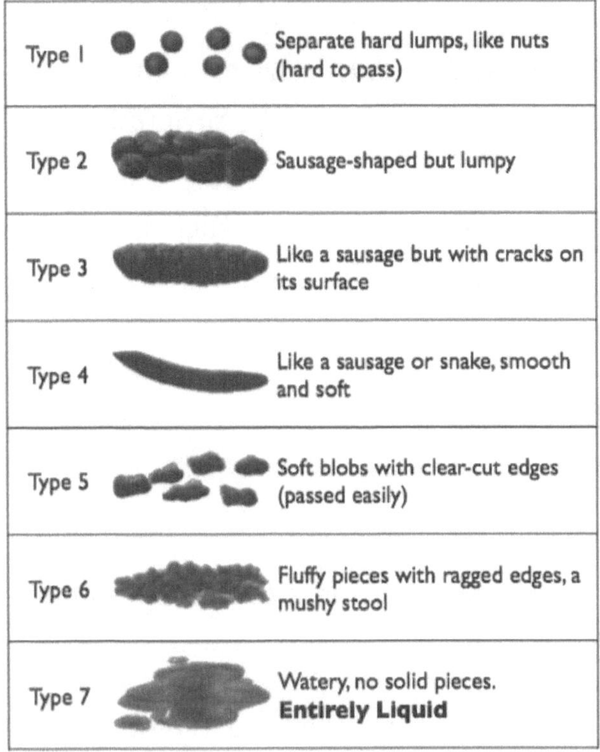

Your respiratory system prevents harmful substances from entering the lungs in three ways. The first line of defense are the small hairs in your nose that act like a filter to keep large particles out. We also have mucus that is produced in the trachea and bronchial tubes that is keeping our air passages moist. This helps grab the dust, bacteria and other harmful substances from entering into the lungs. Finally, the sweeping motion of those tiny little hairs in the trachea, called cilia, keep our air passages clean. When we inhale things like cigarette smoke, those cilia stop working, allowing the toxins into the lungs and damaging the protection we have. Our lungs help detox our bodies, by removing carbonic gases and phlegm. Infectious microbes and other irritants are moved by the blood towards the lungs and we cough it out as phlegm.

Blood is a specialized body fluid. It has four main components: plasma, red blood cells, white blood cells and platelets. Blood has these five main functions:

*transporting oxygen and nutrients to the lungs and tissues

*forming blood clots to prevent too much blood loss

*carrying cells and antibodies that help fight off infection in our bodies

*transporting the waste products to the kidneys and liver

* regulating our body's temperature.

You can see how important all of these functions are to our body's natural ability to detox.

Finally, the lymphatic system works directly with the cardiovascular system to flush toxins out of the body and produce immune cells. It consists of lymph vessels, ducts, nodes and other tissues that work in a manner that is very similar to the way our blood vessels work, except that it is not pumped but rather squeezed through the vessels, when we use our muscles. The lymphatic system is like the sewer system of the body, carrying all the waste from the tissues to the blood stream.

What an incredible system our body is! As we continue in the next chapter, I'll show you what it looks like when we overburden this system.

Chapter Three: What does Toxic Overload Look Like?

You may be asking why if our bodies are so incredibly made, can we even get to a state of overload? It is simple. We are adding more toxins to our body than our system can handle. This is what we refer to as bioaccumulation. Bioaccumulation is the gradual accumulation of substances, such as pesticides or other chemicals, in an organism. Bioaccumulation occurs when an organism absorbs a substance at a rate faster than that at which the substance is lost by catabolism and excretion. Thus, the longer the biological half-life of a toxic substance, the greater the risk of chronic poisoning, even if environmental levels of the toxin are not very high. Bioaccumulation, for example, in fish, can be predicted by models. Hypotheses for molecular size cutoff criteria for use as bioaccumulation potential indicators are not supported by data. Biotransformation can strongly modify bioaccumulation of chemicals in an organism. (Wikipedia, n.d.)

As we live our day to day lives, we are exposing ourselves to toxins. We are breathing them in, digesting them and absorbing them through our skin and our lungs. It is inevitable. Toxins are now in our air, water, soil and food supply. From the time we wake up until we go to bed, we are exposing ourselves to toxins. It begins with the personal care products we are using, to the water we are drinking and bathing in, to all those electronics we use daily in our homes. We find them in our laundry soaps, cleaning products and many of our household items, like furniture, carpets, mattresses and plastics, both in the kitchen and elsewhere, like toys and appliances. The one thing that is certain is that you are exposed to toxins. What is uncertain, is how your body will respond.

As these exposures add up, our body's natural detoxification system gets overloaded. As a result, it can't keep up with the demands on these organs. The toxins can't be released the way they normally are. They then get stored in the cells, muscles and soft tissues of our body. As this accumulation continues, disease sets in. I had no idea how I felt was because I had too many toxins built up in my body. No one had explained any kind of connection between the chronic disease I was suffering from and the role of the environment. Because you are reading this book, I think you may be in the same boat. Some people don't realize how bad they feel, because this accumulation has taken place over many years. You have been adapting to how you feel. It wasn't until I began to remove the toxins, that I truly knew how poorly I had felt. I've seen this to be true for many people that I have helped over the last seven years. It is amazing how we adapt to our health, when the decline is so gradual.

When we begin to build up toxins in our body, we will have symptoms. The number of toxins that are built up, will determine what these symptoms will look like. One of the easiest signs of our overall health, is how we are pooping. It sounds crazy, doesn't it? Remember my Bristol Stool chart from the previous chapter? If we are not eliminating daily, then toxins are building up in your body. What will this look like? It is different for every person. We each have our own unique individual chemistry. No two people will present symptoms the same way. In the beginning, we may notice a change in body odor or a change in our skin. For instance, if we had oily skin and suddenly our skin is very dry. However, if we don't hear our body with these very first symptoms, then there are some pretty good guidelines we can use, indicating that your body is giving you a nudge.

According to Dr. Mark Hyman, (Hyman, n.d.) a practicing family physician and an internationally recognized leader, speaker, educator, and advocate in the field of Functional Medicine, these are the symptoms of chronic toxicity in our body:

- Fatigue
- Muscle aches
- Joint pain
- Sinus congestion
- Postnasal drip
- Excessive sinus problems
- Headaches
- Bloating
- Gas
- Constipation
- Diarrhea
- Foul-smelling stools
- Heartburn

- Sleep Problems

- Difficulty concentrating

- Food cravings

If we don't make changes with these symptoms and the toxins continue to accumulate in our bodies, then we will develop chronic diseases and underlying medical conditions. Our bodies are trying to tell us a story, if we listen.

Chapter Four: Listening to Our Bodies

Do you listen to your body? We all have energy. When that energy is disrupted for any reason, our body sends signals to us. Do you feel your body? Our bodies are always in a state of communication with us. We must learn to identify the signals it gives us, so we can react appropriately.

In the beginning, our body gives us a gentle nudge or a whisper. Hey, I've got something to tell you. Our body will look to get rid of the toxins in any way it can. Some of the very first signs that our body is trying to get rid of toxins, is a change in body odor or excessive oily skin. This is because our body is trying to expel the toxins through our pores. In thinking of the other ways our body eliminates, we may experience diarrhea, sneezing or coughing fits, excessive urination, sore throat, heartburn, nasal congestion or runny nose (from mucus overproduction), or vomiting.

 When we don't listen to those first gentle nudges, then it begins talking a little louder. As the toxins gradually build up in the soft tissue, blood and organs, we may begin experiencing neurological symptoms.

Most people experience fatigue, memory difficulties, sleep impairment, eczema (and other inflammatory conditions, like gout), depression, or "brain fog". As the buildup happens, it damages organs like our kidneys, liver and lungs. These are the key organs that help our bodies to naturally detox.

If we still ignore these signals, then our body starts to scream at us, with the development of chronic diseases and increased rates of brain diseases, including dementia. A chronic disease, if you remember, are symptoms that last a year or more and effect your daily routine. Some chronic diseases are heart disease, diabetes, stroke, high blood pressure, autoimmune diseases, anxiety and depression and different types of cancers.

We want to start feeling our bodies so we can hear the whispers. However, most of us don't listen, until we are at the screaming stage. I know I didn't, because I didn't know what I was dealing with. I had no idea the symptoms I was experiencing were due to toxin exposures in my environment. My first course of action was to go to the doctor. When your body isn't working, that's what we do, right? However, none of the doctors talked to me about toxins in my body or my environment. They didn't talk to me about lifestyle and changes I could make to help myself. Their solution was to treat the symptom, by prescribing medications. These medications were often also causing other problems with my body.

This is a vicious cycle that many of us are on. Unless we are willing to take our hand off the fire, it's not going to get any better. We can't treat a burn, while our hand is still sitting on the oven burner. What I discovered is that when we give our bodies the proper things and remove the toxins, it has the ability to naturally heal itself. Let's take a look at how we can help our body do its job, to detox.

Chapter Five: Detox

Do we really have to subscribe to taking supplements to detox, follow a particular detox diet or cleanse to help our bodies detox? That answer is really unique to each person, depending on how much toxic overload and burden your body is under, and what current health situations you are facing. You have to take your hand off the fire. Remember, our hand keeps burning, if we keep it on the stove. The same holds true for removing the hidden toxins from your home and environment. In order to achieve optimal health, we must remove these toxins. We know that we are not going to get rid of them all; Even I am continuously learning of new detox and cleanse protocols. This is where I know we can make a difference. By not simply treating a symptom, we can actually restore, renew and rejuvenate our health. Do we want to continue to pop pills for our heartburn, or try to find out what is causing the heartburn and eliminate that root cause? In the next chapter, as we go through each pillar of living a toxin free lifestyle, we will explore many of the toxins we want to eliminate. We will focus on ways that we can help our body detox and cleanse now.

There are several ways to help our bodies detox naturally. I will list them and then explain why each of these help our body's natural detoxification system.

1. Limit Alcohol

2. Focus on Sleep

3. Drink More Water

4. Reduce Your Intake of Sugar and Processed Foods

5. Eat Antioxidant Rich Foods

6. Eat Foods High in Prebiotics

7. Reduce Your Salt Intake

8. Increase Your Sweat

Alcohol is one of the most widely consumed substances in the world. It is used by millions of people throughout the United States on a regular basis. Alcohol consumption can have a significant impact on health and well-being. Even light drinking is associated with certain adverse effects. The more alcohol an individual consumes, the greater of an effect it has on their system.

Excessive alcohol use can lead to many health conditions affecting the central nervous system, heart, digestive system, immune system and even our menstrual cycles. (Body Effects, n.d.)

Alcohol is primarily metabolized in your liver, where it is made into acetaldehyde. This is a toxin, that is then converted into acetate, which is a harmful substance that is then removed by our body. When we consume too much alcohol, we can cause damage to the liver functions by causing fat buildup, inflammation and scarring. This is also known as cirrhosis. When this happens, our liver doesn't function as it should. Its ability to remove waste and toxins from the body is compromised.

Sleep is very important to maintain good health and well-being throughout your life. It is important to not only get enough quality sleep but also at the right times. This will help you to protect your mental health, physical health, quality of life and safety.

The way you feel while you're awake, depends in part on what happens while you're sleeping. During sleep, your body is working to support healthy brain function and maintain your physical health. In children and teens, sleep also helps support growth and development. It is a time for our body to heal and nurture itself.

The damage from sleep deficiency can occur instantly (like a car crash), or it can harm you over time. For example, ongoing sleep deficiency can raise your risk for some chronic health problems. It also can affect how well you think, react, work, learn and get along with others. (Sleep deprivation and deficiency, n.d.)

The kidneys act as a natural filtration system for the body, removing waste, toxins and excess water from the blood. The kidneys even cleanse themselves, when the body takes in enough fluid. The kidneys are an integral part of our detox system. In order for them to function properly, we need to make sure we are drinking plenty of water. Water transports waste products through urination, breathing and sweating. It's generally considered healthy to drink half your body weight in ounces of water each day. For instance, if you weigh 150lbs, then you would want to drink 75ounces of water each day.

Sugar and processed Foods have been linked to chronic diseases., like obesity, diabetes, heart disease and even cancer. (Hunger, poor nutrition lead to chronic disease, n.d.) These diseases make it harder for your body to naturally detox itself, because the organs that are vital for this process have been or are being damaged by these diseases. This makes it more difficult for your body to remove toxins.

A great way to help improve the function of the body's natural detox is to eat foods that are high in antioxidants. Antioxidants help fight free radicals and protect the cells. They are the most important thing that we can do to support anti-aging. When our body has too many free radicals, we are in a state known as oxidative stress. Foods like berries, nuts, cocoa and vegetables are high in vitamin A, C, E, selenium, lycopene and lutein which are excellent antioxidants. I found many studies on PubMed.org (so many) on anti-aging. Many of those studies support using foods as our source for antioxidants over supplementation. There is also evidence that as we are looking at our bodies as a whole system, scientists are discovering that aging is reversable and an integrative approach is necessary. There are numerous studies that have proven life extension in simple organisms, but they are still working on translating this to humans. (A Synopsis on Aging-Theories, mechanisms and future prospects, n.d.) This is exciting!

We have to keep the balance of disease-causing bacteria and good bacteria in our digestive system and our microbiome. Antibiotics, poor dental hygiene, use of antibacterial hand soaps and hand sanitizers and some of our food choices can upset this balance and cause many issues for our body, including weakening the immune system. Finding foods that are high in prebiotics/probiotics are a great way to keep a healthy balance. Eating foods like tomatoes, artichokes, bananas, asparagus, onions, garlic and oats are all great sources of prebiotics. Eating fermented foods like kombucha, kimchi, sauerkraut and yogurt can provide probiotics. These foods will help you keep a healthy balance in your microbiome. Using hand sanitizer only when soap and water are unavailable and limiting your use of mouthwash will also help. These products kill all bacteria (both good and bad) and quickly change the balance of your microbiome. The use of antibacterial hand soaps and cleaners are weakening our immune systems, by removing the good bacteria on our skin biome that protect us and are our first line of defense.

When we consume too much salt, our body will begin to retain fluid. This is especially important, if you already have damage to your liver or kidneys. If you feel bloated or have excessive fluid built up, you can drink more water, reduce your sodium and add foods that are rich in potassium. These steps will counterbalance the effect of high sodium levels. Foods like potatoes, squash, beans and bananas are all rich in potassium. Sodium levels are usually very high in packaged food, since it is used as a preservative. Research has found that if you eat too much salt, the extra water stored in your body raises your blood pressure. The more salt you eat, the higher your blood pressure. This places a greater strain on your heart, arteries, kidneys and brain and can lead to heart attacks, strokes, dementia and kidney disease. (National Institute of Health, n.d.)

It is very important to get moving. Exercise has been found to decrease inflammation in the body. Numerous studies and scientific data show that exercise assists the lungs, kidneys, immune system and intestines in becoming more efficient at naturally detoxifying the body. Exercise keeps our body moving, increasing blood circulation and the uptake of oxygen.

This enhances the body's detoxification process. Several studies have found that there is a higher concentration of phthalates, BPA's and heavy metals in sweat than in urine. (Human Elimination of Phthalates: Blood, Urine & Sweat, n.d.) Movement, exercise and activity are great ways to support the natural detoxification of your body.

We now discussed chronic disease, the current state of health in our nation, toxic overload and how to detox naturally. We have discussed the importance of listening to our body, when it gives us signals. We will now learn how to take our hand off the fire.

Chapter Six: The Five Pillars to a Toxin-Free Lifestyle

I developed the five pillars to a toxin-free lifestyle through my own experiences, as well as working with hundreds of individuals and families. My interviews with doctors, experts and industry leaders, confirmed the most important areas to focus on. I have participated in numerous conferences and classes and have researched how we remove toxins from our lifestyle. It will allow us to live our lives with renewed health, focus and energy. If we remove these toxins, we can reduce our chances of succumbing to chronic disease. We must address all five areas and break the toxin free lifestyle down into five pillars. This will make our journey easier and allow us to get our hand off the fire. Renewed health is not possible, unless all five pillars are addressed. Your specific condition will determine where you will start. I focused on one pillar at a time. I am always incorporating new information into my daily routines! The more attention you pay to how your body feels, the easier good choices will be.

In writing this book, I felt that was important to give you the tools that would make an impact in your life. I refer to my toolbox many times. We will all accumulate more tools during our journey. The topic of environmental toxins can become very overwhelming and scary.   Although it can seem frustrating, it is never too late to focus on your health. This toxin free lifestyle is FUN! Removing toxins doesn't mean we can't enjoy great food, look beautiful and have great products. By focusing on our homes and the products you use every day, you will be able to remove the hidden toxins and improve your overall health. As you detox and cleanse your home from these toxins, you will start to see renewed health, better sleep, more focus and more energy. The five pillars of a toxin-free lifestyle are air, water, food, absorption and mental.

There are many more toxins within our homes than I have included in this book. As you continue down your Toxin- Free Lifestyle journey, you may look into more of these. There are toxins in our furniture and the construction materials, we use as well as in many of our appliances. There is also mold that can be found in your homes and offices. However, we will just focus on the five pillars. It is an excellent start and won't be so overwhelming.

Chapter Seven: Air

Were you aware that studies show that the air inside our homes is five times more polluted than the outdoors? This is my number one pillar in living a toxin-free lifestyle. Why is the air inside our homes more toxic than outside? Newer homes are energy efficient, which means they are sealed up tight. The toxic ingredients inside our homes, such as everyday products or construction, furniture and appliances material are staying inside our homes. Many of the newer homes have humidifiers on the heating systems, which can contribute to poor air quality, if not balanced correctly. When the humidity is too high, it allows mold, bacteria and viruses to grow. Low humidity can irritate our eyes, nose and throat and skin.

How many of you use candles, plug-ins or sprays to make your home "smell" better? These items are full of toxins and only masking odors, instead of getting rid of them. The biggest problem has to do with fragrances. Fragrances are considered by many people to be the new second-hand smoke. There are several lawsuits that have been filed seeking to have fragrance-free workplaces. There are many other sources of toxins including cleaning laundry and personal care products. Most of these products have the word fragrance in the ingredient list.

The problem with fragrances is that we don't know what chemicals they contain. This is because fragrances are considered to be a proprietary trade secret. Therefore, companies are not required to disclose what chemicals are included. There are over 3,000 possible chemicals in this one "ingredient". Unscented products are no better, since they contain the same toxins and added chemicals to take away the scent.

In addition to fragrances, there are electronic magnetic frequencies (EMFs). They are created by our smart phones, smart tv's, Wi-Fi routers, microwaves and other appliances and power lines around our homes. Our bodies have a frequency. The higher the frequency, the healthier we are. When our frequencies are lowered by toxins, we begin to get sick. The EMF's disrupt these frequencies and can confuse our bodies. This results in damage to our cells and affects the function of our nervous system. Very high exposures can even result in the development of unusual growths and cancer. However, the most common symptoms of EMF toxicity are sleep disturbances, including insomnia. (Current Health Effects, n.d.)

Flame retardants were developed in the 1970's to prevent or slow down the growth of a fire. They are often added or applied to the following products:

- Furnishings, such as foam, upholstery, mattresses, carpets, curtains and fabric blinds.

- Electronics and electrical devices, such as computers, laptops, phones, televisions, and household appliances, as well as wires and cables.

- Building and construction materials, including electrical wires and cables, and insulation materials, such as polystyrene and polyurethane insulation foams.

- Transportation products, such as seats, seat covers and fillings, bumpers, overhead compartments, and other parts of automobiles, airplanes, and trains.

According the National Institute of Environmental Health and Sciences, many flame retardants have been removed from the market or are no longer produced. However, because they do not break down easily, they can remain in the environment for years. They can also bioaccumulate or build up in people and animals over time, causing health issues like disruption of the endocrine and immune systems, toxicity to the reproductive system, cancer, impaired neurologic function and adverse effects on fetal and child development. A study conducted by the Environmental Working Group commissioned five separate laboratories to study the blood from umbilical cords. They found 232 chemicals and flame retardants ingredients that haven't been used in the United States since 2005 in all samples. (EWG.ORG, n.d.)

Construction materials like carpet, paint and plastics found in our electronics fare loaded with many toxins, ranging from asbestos to lead and formaldehyde.

Over 90,000 people worldwide die each year from asbestos-related illnesses. (Asbestos, n.d.) Exposure to asbestos can lead to lung diseases, including mesothelioma, which is a form of lung cancer. Asbestos can be found in floor tiles, pipes and roofing shingles.

Formaldehyde is a known carcinogen according to the <u>World Health Organization</u>(WHO). It was grandfathered in under the original 1976 version of the TSCA (Toxic Substances Control Act). Therefore, it has never been fully assessed by the EPA. It is an irritant to the thin tissue membranes inside your nose, other respiratory passages and inside your gut. Long term exposure can cause asthma-like respiratory problems and skin irritation, such as dermatitis and itching.

It is found in polymers that are used in plywood and carpet manufacturing, resins important to paper product manufacturing and polyurethane foam insulation manufacturing.

There are many things that are in the air we breathe every single day. That is why the air in our homes is more polluted than the outdoors. Let me leave you with some good news and give you just a couple tips that will help you get started. One step is to purchase products that are fragrance-free or do not have any synthetic fragrances. We do not sleep with electronics in the bedroom. In my office, I am direct-wired into my computer rather than using wi-fi. I always make sure the wi-fi is turned off at night and keep the router placed a safe distance away from where we congregate in the home. As I have continued our journey, I have been making better choices for the materials we use in our home and look for safer options.

Are you ready for the next pillar?

Chapter Eight: Water

Our water supplies are contaminated with many different chemicals that are toxic to our bodies. These chemicals get into our water supplies through the air, runoff from farming and waste from factories. They also become contaminated through our own personal use. For instance, if we flush pharmaceuticals down the toilet, they remain in the water supply and are very hard to break down and filter out. Chemicals that have been banned for use in the United States are often still being used in other parts of the world. As a result, they are re-entering our water sources. Did you know that when a chemical is banned within the United States, it is often sold to other countries? That just feels so wrong. Depending on where you are, will determine your exposure to those chemicals. We will first look at some of the most common toxins that are found in our water supply.

Heavy metals like lead, mercury, aluminum, arsenic and cadmium are usually found in water in trace amounts. However, even these amounts can be toxic to humans. Heavy metals become toxic when they accumulate in the soft tissue of our body and are more difficult for us to expel. Natural and human activities are contaminating the environment and its resources. They are discharging more toxins, than the environment can handle. According to a PubMed study, these metals are systemic toxicants known to cause adverse health effects in humans, including cardiovascular diseases, developmental abnormalities, neurologic and neurobehavioral disorders, diabetes, hearing loss, hematologic and immunologic disorders, and various types of cancer. (Heavy Metals Toxicity and the Environment, n.d.)

Fluoride is added to many of our water sources, since it was once thought to be beneficial for our oral health. However, studies show that fluoride is a neurotoxin. It does not prevent tooth decay, as was once thought. A PubMed study found that the addition of fluoride to the world's water supply and the widespread use of aluminum in vaccinations for infants and young children, alone or as aluminofluoride can result in immunoexcitotoxicity that can lead to the pathological changes seen in ASD (Autism Spectrum Disorder) (Immunoexcitotoxicity as the central mechanism of etiopathology and treatment of autism spectrum disorders: A possible role of fluoride and aluminum, n.d.)

Chlorine and chloramines are chemicals that are added to a water source to sanitize the water. Although the Environmental Protection Agency considers these chemicals to be safe for use in drinking water and bathing water, they can irritate the skin and respiratory system. Once I began filtering that out of our water sources, I could still taste and smell it at restaurants or hotels.

Pesticides have been widely found in our drinking water. They come from agricultural areas through rivers, lakes streams and even rain. These pesticides can also come from our own lawns and gardens and enter the water supply. In my research for this book, I found out that the EPA regulates many of the contaminants in water. However, many pesticides are not regulated contaminants. I found that the regulatory agencies which are supposed to be protecting us are letting us down. The Environmental Working Group has a website where you can get the water safety test for your zip code. (TapWater Database, n.d.) I found that my water supply had 24 contaminants, with eight that exceeded EWG's health guidelines. This is why it is necessary for you to do your own research into the quality of your drinking water.

Pesticides have various health risks and with different levels depending on the type of pesticide. Some of the main health concerns are organ toxicity, reproductive toxicity and even cancer. There have been many lawsuits over Roundup which uses glyphosate in their pesticide. This ingredient has been linked to non-Hodgkin's lymphoma. As of this writing, over <u>52,000 U.S. lawsuits</u>—and counting—have been filed on behalf of agricultural laborers, gardeners, and others diagnosed with non-Hodgkin's lymphoma after being exposed to Roundup. Bayer, which acquired Monsanto in 2018, has lost all three Roundup lawsuits that went to trial. The juries have delivered verdicts of $289 million, $80 million, and $2 billion. (Class Action Lawsuit, n.d.)

It is also important that we bathe in clean water. There are some experts who suggest this is even more important than your drinking water. This is because the pores on your skin are opened by the heat of the water, which allows the toxicants to be absorbed directly into your body. The EWG recommends some great water filtration systems. What I have found to be best is reverse osmosis. I highly encourage you to consider a whole house system. However, I do understand that this may not be feasible for everyone. In that case, make sure to find good filtration for both your drinking and bathing water. There are some great filters that can be installed on your shower head. There is excellent information on water in Bobbi Schaben's story in Chapter Twelve.

We will look at the top offenders that we absorb through our skin in the next pillar.

Chapter Nine: Absorb

When most people (including myself) hear healthy lifestyle, they think about their diet and exercise.   I did not know that many of the items I was using inside my home were actually poisoning me. This is one of my favorite topics. Most people are not aware that we absorb many toxins every day. It is one of the biggest "aha" moments that many people have.

 Our skin is the body's largest organ. It is part of our body's natural detox process. Studies have shown that products that we put on our skin can be detected in the blood within minutes. According to the CDC, dermal absorption is the transport of a chemical from the outer surface of the skin both into the skin and into the body. The absorption of chemicals through the skin can occur without being noticed. The rate of dermal absorption depends primarily on the outer layer of the skin called the *stratum corneum* (SC). The SC serves an important barrier function, by keeping molecules from passing into and out of the skin. It, therefore, protects the lower layers of the skin. The extent of absorption is dependent on the following factors:

- Skin integrity (damaged vs. intact)

- Location of exposure (thickness and water content of the stratum corneum; skin temperature)

- Physical and chemical properties of the hazardous substance

- Concentration of a chemical on the skin surface

- Duration of exposure

- The surface area of skin exposed to a hazardous substance (Skin Exposure and Effects, n.d.)

Chemicals that we apply to our bodies are also found in our cells. One study found that parabens can stimulate the growth of certain types of breast cancer. They have been found in both breast tissue and breast cancer tumors. (Breast Cancer & Parabens, n.d.) Another study on EWG's website found over 200 chemicals in the blood of unborn babies! What? They have already been exposed before birth. The chemicals found included: parabens, phthalates and 1,4 Dioxane. This study emphasized the importance of being aware of what we put into our bodies.

There have been no changes to the chemical regulations for skin care and personal care products for over 80 years. Although most people assume that the federal government regulates the safety of our personal care products, that is not actually true. This is reflected in the following statement on the FDA's website: Companies and individuals who manufacture or market cosmetics have a legal responsibility to ensure the safety of their products. Neither the law nor FDA regulations require specific tests to demonstrate the safety of individual products or ingredients. The law also does not require cosmetic companies to share their safety information with the FDA. (Authority over Cosmetics, n.d.)

More than 40 nations worldwide have enacted regulations specifically targeting the safety and ingredients of cosmetics and personal care products. Some of these nations have restricted or completely banned more than 1,400 chemicals from cosmetic products. By contrast, the U.S. Food and Drug Administration has banned or restricted only nine chemicals for safety reasons. (Cosmetic Safety, n.d.)

From the over 85,000 chemicals used in our products, less than 1% have been tested for safety. There have been no changes to our laws governing toxic exposure since 1938. However, a new bill called The Personal Care Product Safety Act was reintroduced in 2019.

For these reasons, it is important to take our personal health into our own hands. YOU are your best advocate. We cannot depend on someone else to protect us. Our government is not necessarily concerned about our best interests.

This is why I trust the information that is available from the Environmental Working Group. They are an organization that conducts research into the safety of our products. They also help to promote legislation that protects consumers. Their website is full of very useful information, which I recommend that you look at. It is: www.EWG.org.

The Safe Cosmetics organization does fantastic research on personal care products. They also work on developing legislation to protect consumer safety. They can be found at: www.safecosmetics.org

It was very important for me to start reading labels. I was able to determine the ingredients in the products and whether they had any harmful side effects. I would look at an ingredient and then research any potential dangers. Based on my research, I determined that I wanted to avoid parabens, phthalates, sodium laurel sulfate and fragrances. These ingredients have been found to cause damage to internal organs, disrupt our endocrine system, cause skin and lung irritation, and even cancer. These ingredients can be found in shampoo, conditioners, body wash, lotion, skin care and beauty care products, as well as laundry products, cleaning products, dish soaps and dishwashing detergent.   These are things that we use every day.

If you don't have the time to do extensive research, there are two useful apps that you can download to your phone. They are Healthy Living by the Environmental Working Group and the other is Think Dirty. There is no cost to download these apps, which are updated frequently. How about an EASY button? I personally order all my safe products through a company that I know and trust. I know their standards, have gone to their farms and laboratories and have talked with their scientists. I don't have to read the labels, and my everyday products for our home are delivered right to my doorstep. Here's a link so you can check them out: http://aimeecarlson.com/start

All of this information can be overwhelming at first. The important thing to remember is to take a step at a time. It is not necessary to change everything immediately. You can just take one small step today. Our next chapter will cover food. That was a hard one for me.

Chapter Ten: Food

"Let food be thy medicine, and medicine be thy food."
This quote is attributed to Hippocrates. However,
some studies show this actual quote cannot be found
in his writings. However, Hippocrates did consider
nutrition one of the main tools that a doctor can use.
We now have a hard time finding physicians who are
willing to address illness with their patients, by talking
about diet and lifestyle. The common theme is to
prescribe medications and treatments that put a band
aid on the symptom, rather than get to the root of the
problem. Please don't misunderstand me. I do believe
there are situations where physicians are necessary.
Each person should make their own choices here. You
know which lifestyle changes you are willing to make.
The right foods AND clean foods have the power to
heal our bodies. At the same time, the wrong foods
are contributing to inflammation and disease in the
body.

 There are several toxins that we want to avoid in our
food. The number one toxin to avoid are pesticides.
We have already discussed the lawsuits involving
Roundup. Roundup is a pesticide known as

glyphosate. It is a known carcinogen that is still widely applied to our food sources during the farming process. It is also used in many homes. Studies show that glyphosates can be found in every single person. That should scare you! Over 1 billion pounds of pesticides are used in the United States (US) each year and approximately 5.6 billion pounds are used worldwide. (Pesticide Use and Exposure Worldwide, n.d.)

Each type of pesticide has a different effect on our bodies. Insecticides tend to be more toxic to humans, and the amount and exposure of the pesticide determines its toxicity We can swallow, inhale or come into direct skin contact with pesticides from drinking contaminated water, eating treated food and direct exposure in parks, lawns and lakes. Pesticides have been proven to cause reproductive and developmental effects, cancer, kidney and liver damage and endocrine disruption. Children, whose bodies are still developing, are particularly vulnerable. They are exposed to pesticides at home, daycare, schools and playgrounds. Children are more likely to crawl on the ground and put their contaminated hands in their mouths.

Research shows that children are even exposed to pesticides in utero.

These are the reasons I do a couple of things in our home. First, I purchase organic produce. Since many of you are working within a budget, there are a few useful resources. It is easiest to purchase the organic foods that you eat the most. Second, you can check out the clean 15 and dirty dozen at www.ewg.org. I also like to use an effective cleaner with all my produce. I like the Thieves Fruit and Veggie Soak. It is highly concentrated, so I use one capful for a full sink of cold water. It gently removes pesticide residue, wax, dirt and debris. It also helps my produce to last longer Fruit & Veggie Soak

Another important toxin in foods are genetically modified foods or GMO's. These are also being referred to on our labels as engineered foods or bioengineered foods. Genetically modified foods are produced from organisms that have changes introduced into their DNA through genetic engineering. In the United States, products do not have to label their ingredients as genetically modified. The Dark Act is the start of GMO labeling in the United

States. However, it is far from the protection that consumers deserve. It requires that some – but not all- GMO's must be labeled in the United States by 2022.

There have not been any long-term safety studies on GMO's. However, initial studies have shown that some potential health risks are allergic reactions, antibiotic resistance, immune-suppression, loss of nutrition and cancer. The Center for Food Safety (GMO Search, n.d.) has compiled a shopping guide to help you avoid GMO's in your food. They list the "Big Five" foods to avoid, which are corn, soybeans, canola, cottonseed and sugar beets used in processed foods. Our meat, while not genetically modified (yet) is fed with genetically modified grain. GMOs also enter into food in the form of processed crop derivatives and inputs derived from other forms of genetic engineering, such as synthetic biology. Some examples include hydrolyzed vegetable protein corn syrup, molasses, sucrose, textured vegetable protein, flavorings, vitamins, yeast products, microbes and enzymes, flavors, oils and fats, proteins, and sweeteners. Another great resource on this topic is the NonGMO Project. (Americans Deserve Better, n.d.)

Another reason to stay away from processed foods are the preservatives that are used. Sodium benzoate is a common food preservative used in processed foods and drinks to prevent spoilage. Food labels will list this as sodium benzoate. However, it could also be listed as benzoic acid, potassium benzoate or benzoate. This preservative has been linked to hyperactivity in children.

Sodium nitrite is usually found in meat products like sausage, cured meats, canned meats and lunch meats. You can find it labeled as sodium nitrite, sodium nitrate or nitrite. This preservative can damage cells and morph into molecules that can cause cancer.

Sodium sulfite is used in wines and dried fruits. According to the FDA (Food and Drug Administration) approximately one in 100 people have a sensitivity to this ingredient. Most of these people also suffer from asthma, but can present as headaches, breathing problems and rashes. In severe cases, it can completely close the airways, leading to death by cardiac arrest.

Sulfur dioxide can be found in beer, soft drinks, wine, dried fruits, vinegar and potato products. The FDA has banned their use on raw fruits and vegetables, because of the toxicity of sulfur. However, it is still allowed in the other products. It causes bronchial issues, rashes and destroys vitamins B1 and E. It is not recommended for consumption by children.

The last preservative is propyl paraben, which is used in bread products and tortillas, as well as food dyes. Because of cross contamination, it is now showing up in beverages, dairy products, meats and vegetables. One study found methyl, ethyl and propyl parabens in 90% of over 267 food items purchased in the United States. (Khetan) This preservative is a known endocrine disruptor. It has been shown to decrease sperm counts and has altered the expression of genes, especially those found in breast cancer cells. It actually accelerates the growth of the cancerous cells. Some alternative names used on labels are propyl paraben, propyl p-hydroxybenzoate and propyl Para hydroxybenzoate.

We can also find things in processed foods that are truly toxic to our bodies, like additives, artificial sweeteners, food coloring and dyes and hydrogenated fats. Many people in the health and wellness space refer to these highly processed foods as "frankinfoods." They have no nutritional value. They can cause more harm, by producing free radicals in our body. Did you know that many European nations have banned many of these ingredients? However, in the United States they are still allowed. Companies like Heinz and Quaker Oats actually have two very different products that are sold in European nations versus what is packaged and sold on our shelves in the United States. It even varies from state to state.

 What is left to eat? How do we make sure we are not allowing these toxins into our meals? What I did in the beginning was turn those labels around. I needed to not just look at nutritional content, like calories, fat, sugar or sodium levels. It is also necessary to look at the ingredients. I, therefore, made a rule of thumb that if there were more than five ingredients, it didn't go in my cart. By doing this, I knew that I was eliminating most of the toxins listed above. After acclimating ourselves to this, I took it a step further and switched to whole foods. I no longer shopped up and down the aisles. I limited my visits to the perimeters of the grocery stores. I made sure that I was purchasing organic fruit and vegetables, especially for the dirty dozen. I am still far from perfect. Food has been one of the hardest hurdles for me on this toxin-free lifestyle. I toyed with eating healthy for the first five years. I would eat really well for a week or so and then drop off the wagon. I'd use every excuse in the book including I was traveling, I was busy, or I hadn't been to the store. The real problem was that I wasn't making my health a priority. This past year, I have been taking baby steps toward living a more plant-based lifestyle. I have found that I feel great. It makes my body perform its best. I encourage you to figure out what works best for you and your body. There are many ways to eat as a lifestyle. I did not use the word diet. I don't believe in diets. It is my opinion that you will not see lasting results, unless you incorporate lifestyle changes. I also don't believe that there is one answer that fits all. When you start really paying attention to your body, you will be able to tell if you have any food sensitivities and what makes you feel the most energized. I found that dairy and iceberg lettuce were a definite no for me.

"There is not a fix for everybody, it's what works for your body!" Aimee Carlson, The Toxin Terminator

Chapter Eleven: Mental

The last pillar that we will discuss in living a natural lifestyle is the emotional and mental pillar. I strongly believe this may be the most important pillar of all. There are two branches to this pillar. There are external, internal and physical mental and emotional toxins. We will examine each of them.

External toxins are the easiest to talk about. They involve the negative energy that are created in your life by the relationships around you. Do you find yourself feeling exhausted after spending time with someone? We all have people in our lives who always seem to bring us down. It is toxic. These people may be doing more than just emotionally bringing us down. It is important to remember that God created you for beautiful things and you deserve more. I hope that you feel this inside and find the courage to change your circumstances. These external toxins are the drama that is caused by family and friends. These are the easiest types of toxins to distance ourselves from. However, sometimes we are in relationships where the toxins have evolved into physical or emotional abuse. If this applies to you or someone you know, check out my good friend Heather Knight's podcast "Surviving to Thriving." Heather discusses domestic violence and gives you the tools to succeed in life.

It is sometimes easy for us to remove ourselves from these toxin relationships, while other times it is not. We might not feel good enough about ourselves to expect to be treated better than what we are. These may be people in our family. While it is not possible for me to make decisions for you, I do want to empower you. You do have a choice and you matter.

Internal toxins are my favorite to talk about. It has been the biggest transformation in my life, and I know it can also be for you. When we realize that we have choices and our words have meaning, we can begin to have the transformation occur.

Our brains do not know the difference between what is real and what is not. For example, we have all gone to or watched a movie. How many times have you cried, or jumped from fear or surprise?   It is a movie, with actors playing out a scene on the screen in front of you. It's not real. However, you have a very real physical reaction.

How about this one? You have a conversation (OK, argument) with someone. You re-live every word of that argument over and over again. This conversation is now happening thousands of times. You are not able to forgive that person, because you hang on to it. We are forming a groove in our brain and we are establishing a pattern. Even though the conversation happened only once, you are keeping it in your mind, by reliving the words that were exchanged. This happened to me a lot.   Since this was the focus of my energy, I wasn't able to forgive and move on. This damaged many relationships in my life.

These grooves were often formed by other people in our lives. They could be people who are influential to us, such as a parent, teacher or mentor. The words they repeated became grooves for you. They could also have been words or thoughts about yourself, such as "I'm so stupid", or I'm so forgetful", or "I'm always late". Our brain interprets these thoughts as reality. We then become the person who is always late or the forgetful one. Many women say things about one of their physical features. This could be I don't like my hair, my nose, my legs, etc. If you keep repeating these things, you will start to view yourself as ugly and not pretty. It will eventually become your reality. You stop doing your hair, wearing make-up or even trying to feel beautiful on the outside.

These words become our reality. We are creating on the outside, what we are thinking. If you repeat harsh words, negative encounters and focus on the negative, that is what your reality will be. I believe that we can manifest our realities. This is reflected in my experience from many years ago. The franchise I was in, had a nationwide contest to find the best five-person team. It involved a year-long process of competitions and training with our crews. At the time, I owned five different locations. When the competition was announced, I told my administrative team that we would have the winning team. I told our teams this throughout the entire process. I had them envision competing at the national competition and walking on the stage to receive their $10,000 award. While at the conference, I even introduced myself as the franchisee with the All-Star National Champions. I had been in the organization at the time for 30 years, so I knew everyone. I was choosing the words to speak. On the night of the awards, our team won. This is one of many examples in my life that the power of my words, dictated my thoughts, to create my actions and create my reality. It really works.

It is also possible to create new grooves. You can decide to change the words you use, which change the thoughts and actions that you take.   I go back to the Bible on this one. Look at what the bible says about our words, Proverbs 15:4 "Gentle words bring life and health; a deceitful tongue crushes the spirit." Proverbs 18:4 says "A person's words can be life-giving water; words of true wisdom are as refreshing as a bubbling brook. My favorite is Philippians 4:8 "Finally, brethren, whatsoever things are true, whatsoever things *are* honest, whatsoever things *are* just, whatsoever things *are* pure, whatsoever things *are* lovely, whatsoever things *are* of good report; if *there be* any virtue, and if *there be* any praise, think on these things".

The most recent thing I learned, which was very important for me, is that feelings are just feelings. They are neither right nor wrong, good or bad. This was very empowering for me. I grew up thinking there were good feelings like happy and joyous and bad feelings like sadness and anger. I was taught that you only displayed the good ones. It is a relief to know that isn't true. Feelings are there to feel fully and release. Sometimes, there isn't a reason for us to have a particular feeling.   That knowledge made me free. When we are looking for a reason for the feeling, aren't we really looking for something or someone to blame?

What is the physical effect on our bodies when we have these emotional toxins? If we keep ourselves in a constant state of negativity, our bodies stay in a fight or flight mode. This adds considerable stress to our bodies. We can actually create illness by being in this state of oxidative stress. It is where our bodies are creating too many free radicals and our body cannot detoxify their harmful effects with antioxidants. Oxidative stress can damage cells, proteins and DNA, which contribute to aging. Many people refer to oxidative stress as the silent or secret killer. This is because we don't see stress, we just see the effect that it has on the body. We must learn good stress relieving tools and what we can do to increase the antioxidants in the body.

My top three things for reducing stress are prayer, journaling and meditation. Prayer reminds me who is in charge. When I am feeling stressed, it is often because I am trying to control a situation. When I pray, I am reminded that I am not in the driver's seat. His plan for me is much bigger and better than I could even imagine. Journaling helps me get the thoughts out of my head and onto paper, where I can then release it. Before I started using this tool, my thoughts were very negative. My husband and I incorporated the Stop, Drop and Roll technique. In grade school, they taught you that if you were on fire, you should stop, drop and roll. When my brain was on fire and when I would get into my grooves, I would literally stop, drop to the ground and roll. It was the only thing I could do to stop the thoughts. We now think that it was pretty funny, but it worked. I didn't have to do it for a long time. I only did it long enough for me to start recognizing my patterns. You will also find what works for you.

Meditation was a very hard modality for me to learn. I struggled to quiet my mind. It was even difficult for me to sit still for even five minutes. However, that was OK. I didn't have to be quiet in the beginning. I just needed to complete the meditation. Over time, I learned to channel and quiet my thoughts. It is now a tool that I really enjoy.

Scientists are now discovering more about the gut/brain connection. They are learning that the gut is truly a second brain. Much of the communication is happening from the gut TO the brain, not the other way around. This happens through the vagus nerve. We also have neurotransmitters in the brain that control our feelings and emotions. Scientists are now finding that our microbiome has a direct effect on our emotions. Therefore, what we eat, and the health of our digestive system is crucial to our overall emotional and mental health.

Inflammation can occur for many reasons. However, when our digestive system is inflamed, our brain is too. The inflammation can cause us to experience depression, anxiety, sadness, frustration and anger. By balancing the disease-causing bacteria and the beneficial bacteria, scientists show that we can actually alter the brain's chemistry of the brain. As a result, it can affect our moods and emotions. There are certainly pre and probiotics that can balance our microbiome. This also applies to eating fermented foods that are high in probiotics like sauerkraut, yogurt, kombucha, kimchi and kefir. In addition to balancing the microbiome, we must ensure that we have the proper minerals and enzymes to properly digest our foods. If we do this, it will eliminate the inflammation. I know that before I started to use supplements, I struggled to eliminate bloating and excess gas. I am sure that this affected my stress levels. It is been repeatedly demonstrated that people who suffer from anxiety and depression have been able to change their diets and find relief from the symptoms that had plagued them for years.

Chapter Twelve: Incredible Stories of Recovery

The following chapter has stories from these beautiful ladies that have come into my life through my podcast, The Toxin Terminator. They have had a great impact on me. Each of these women share their experience with chronic disease, how that was manifesting in their lives, what they did and, most importantly, how their life is now. I believe stories to be the connectors with us. We derive true understanding by listening to the stories of others. Some of you may be going through the same experience and some are not. However, we can learn from each one. It is a great honor to be able to share once again their beautiful stories. Let's see how all this works together.

Libby Wright

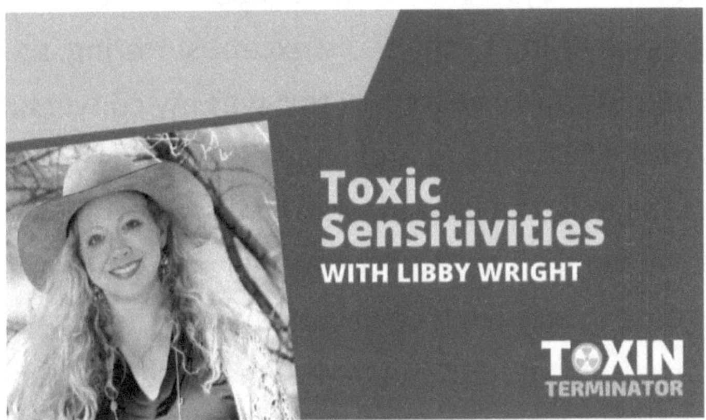

"It was a long journey of 10 years to get to the Lyme diagnosis. It started after my fourth child. I just got really sick, I was 30 and I had about a two-year period where I had difficulty even walking across the room. I wasn't sleeping well, and my bedpost was my IV holder. This was because I couldn't absorb nutrition, so I was getting IV nutrients. I had a fever every day for almost two years. Once the doctors finally figured out what was going on, they compared my pain to that of undiagnosed and untreated cancer pain. It was significant and it was really challenging. I would get my kids down to bed at night. I would then lay on the couch, because I couldn't even lay next to my husband and I would pray and cry. I would say God, I think this is killing me, I think it is killing my family. Everywhere I go, they give me this diagnosis and some more pills. It doesn't help, it just makes me worse. I don't think I'm bringing anything to the table except suffering, so just take me. At thirty years old, this was my conversation with God. My husband and I had discussions about if I didn't make it, the kind of woman that I would want to raise my family. This was because I really didn't think I was going to survive. The second half of that prayer was always if you don't take me, then use me. I wanted to use this experience for some kind of good. Don't waste this experience. Therefore, it was a lot of trial and error. My husband was actually an OBGYN at the time and finally after another round of specialists all over the country, he said that he couldn't just sit there and watch me die. He said that he had to do something about it. He started looking into functional medicine. He actually went back to school and got certified in functional and integrative medicine. At his first conference he called me after an hour, and said I think I know how to get you well. He worked diligently and he did get me well.

I had an underlying genetic condition that we didn't understand. Therefore, if I could go back and look at it that would have been important. The chronic inflammatory response syndrome occurs when you get very sick from mold bio toxins in water damaged buildings. It's not the same type of mold that you would see growing in your shower. It is mold that would develop after flooding or in your air conditioning vents. It can be located anywhere. My body doesn't have a way to get rid of it. As a result, toxins were constantly building up. We are living in a very toxic world. There are hits coming everywhere from environmental toxins with the mold biotoxin, chemical sensitivities and food that is just not really food. Someone 300 years ago wouldn't recognize most of what we eat today. When you combine this with electromagnetic sensitivity to Wi-Fi, appliances and cell phones, it is no wonder why so many people have chronic illness. Therefore, it's probably not just one thing. Many people get tick bites. Some of them get tested for Lyme and it shows that they have Lyme. However, they don't have any symptoms. It is like having a bucket that gets filled up with toxicity. The bucket starts overflowing and seeps into every corner of our lives. That is when there is a problem. So, What I would tell myself 10 or 20 years ago is that we have to find a way to detoxify every corner of your life, because that is how we will prevent this. That is when the healing can really begin. Many of the people I work with have kicked Lyme disease. They have overcome serious autoimmune problems but they're still not completely well. The reason why I can't get well isn't a mystery. It is because of the toxic environment. We need to look inside of our homes.

Due to the MHTFR gene mutation, my body does not process toxins in the same was as someone who does not have this gene mutation. As the buckets fill up, they keep recycling in my body rather than being expelled through normal detoxification methods. This is a major reason why me and my children got sick. The symptoms vary based on what the person's weaknesses are. For some people it might be a migraine. For others, it could be gut health issues or joint pain. My whole family has it. Each person's symptoms are different based on their area of weakness. I have one child who is a gymnast, whose major issue is her joints.

I was like the Canary in the coal mine. I was the first one who experienced symptoms. Looking back on it, the problems that I had, such as headaches or stomach

pain were due to the Lyme Disease. At the time, I am
screaming that we have to deal with this situation.
You could not hit the ignore button on what was going
on with me. I was working with some great specialists.
The interesting thing about Lyme is that it is an
infection. I am not completely against western
medicine. There is a role for it. I needed to get rid of
the infections. However, the antibiotics were not
enough. They caused their own set of problems
because of all the toxicity. Antibiotics don't just kill off
the bad stuff. They also kill off the good stuff. The first
thing that we focused on was my diet. I had adopted
the standard American diet. The one thing with chronic
illness that I talk about, is the thing that you have the
least amount of energy for, is what you need to focus
on the most. You need to find a way through it. It is
usually your diet. It is very easy to say, I'll just go
through the drive through or I'll just buy this
convenience food. The next thing we know is we're
loaded down with food toxins. The first thing I did was
get rid of the sodas and then the processed foods. My
husband Jamie is a physician. We've done a lot of
curriculum writing together. He has a 150-year rule.
The rule is if it wasn't around 150 years ago, you

shouldn't eat it. There were no Twinkies 150 years ago. I don't know where the Twinkie tree is. It's an interesting methodology that we've developed. We have used it with our Fortune 500 company clients and private patients. My husbands' practice has changed from traditional OB GYN and surgery to integrative wellness.

 One of the things that we learned, was that we needed to educate people on how to detoxify with food. It was a lost art form. Nobody knows how to eat the foods that God designed for our bodies. Changing your food is one of the biggest things that you can do to make a huge impact on your body. I actually did a challenge with our corporate wellness clients at least once a year, where we would time how long it would take to make something unhealthy versus something healthy. We always found that the real convenience food was something healthy. You can stick your hand in a bag of almonds pull it out and you have breakfast. Another objection I would often get is that it's too expensive to eat like that. I would do a challenge with my corporate people every year. We would set up a weekend's worth of meals for a family with the standard American diet and compare it to the way we eat as a family. It was always about 20 to 30% less expensive to eat the way that we do. I learned that when we eat the standard American diet, we're not nourishing ourselves. As a result, the hunger is always there. The reason why we are still hungry even if we just ate a Big Mac, fries and a Coke and we can't physically fit anymore in our stomach. Why do we still feel hungry? It is because our body is still telling us that it needs to be nourished. This is very important for people who are losing weight. If you nourish yourself, it takes care of itself.

We, therefore, looked at food as one of the first things within our home. Water quality was also very important to us. I recently moved to Arizona and love many things about it. However, the water is so chlorinated it is almost like pool water. It is very different from the well water that I was used to in Michigan. The quality of the water was our top priority. We need to make sure that is hydrating effectively. This is because not all water is equal. If you switch over to a high-quality water, it will improve your health.

Since I home school my children, I wanted to include them on this health journey.   I wanted to equip them for their lives. When they are on their own, they will already have been exposed to these ideas and understand them.   Our daughter just turned 15 and loves makeup. However, I would not let her buy commercial makeup with all the bad ingredients. She did a school science project a couple years ago. She actually created her own line of chap sticks and lotion based on what she learned.   My daughter is very religious about checking the labels. I presented the information to her. She got to experience it herself and understand why what we're putting on our skin, the largest organ of our body, is so important. This has been ignored for a long time by the medical community. We use many essential oils, especially those which have been shown to help with mold biotoxin. Therefore, we diffuse essential oils in our home.

I was diagnosed with advanced stage neurologic Lyme disease in 2013. The nurse practitioner told me, "I have never seen anyone this sick before. Your immune system looks like someone who is in the hospital actively dying of AIDS. Your body is shutting down and you're not going to survive this, if you don't take really radical action." I took that very hard because I had already been through so much. This has included interstitial cystitis and Graves' disease with heart involvement. I wondered how I was going to cope with something else. She told me that it was like cancer. If I didn't treat it like cancer, I wasn't going to survive. You need to quit your job. You need to get a nanny for the kids, and you need to lay down. It is necessary to focus on this until you get well. She said that she thought they would be able to get me well.

I was feeling overwhelmed. I asked why to bother to fight this because something else is going to pop up. It made me feel that I just couldn't do it anymore. It made me feel like overwhelming pain was the story of my life. What is the point in fighting? However, I took a moment and reflected. I did a silent prayer to God. I remember seeing the equation, OP=OP. It meant that overwhelming pain equals more overwhelming pain. At this point, a second avenue opened up in my mind. What if overwhelming pain could equal overcoming power? What if that could be my equation? In that moment, I decided that if it was at all within my power, I was going to take this overwhelming pain and turn it into something good and have it become overwhelming power.   Having the right mindset is a major part of recovery. We must get rid of the bad to bring in the good. It is a toxicity that isn't talked about often enough, especially in the chronic illness community. The doctors, God love them, are wonderful. However, they've got their diagnosis code or their pill. If they're more alternative minded, it might be acupuncture or an herb. That is all wonderful. However, if we don't have our minds under control, it's going to be hard to win any battle. I was interviewed by a well-known nurse psychiatrist about a year ago. He said if I hadn't had that mindset, I wouldn't have survived. I believe that is true.

 I remember thinking, how am I going to do this? I had always wanted to write a book. During this time, I wrote a book on stress called the Art of Worry. This is because we're all master meditators. We either meditate on the positive or on the negative. Meditating on the negative is worry. We are all very good at that. It's about retraining our mind, our spirit and our soul to ask how we can turn this around. How can we find the positive? It is not about being a Pollyanna, we need to be real about it. If you look at

Psalms, King David would lament the horrible things that had happened to him. I have always loved one of the concepts that I teach in revolutionary joy, which is to complain like a King. You can complain and talk about whatever you want. Our only rule is that at the end of the complaint, you must discover a way to find joy or something positive to come out of this moment. We cannot be stuck left focusing on the negative. If we do that, we get in a very nasty loop. That is probably the worst possible toxin we could ever encounter.

During this time, our son had Lyme Disease and co-infections and our daughter was very sick and getting frequent fevers at school. We couldn't figure out why. I had sent her to school as part of my plan to take care of myself. However, they kept sending her home. It turned out to be a gluten sensitivity. She was getting gluten in her lunch and I didn't realize it. When my daughter was very young, she would sit, and cry. I was determined that even if I had to crawl to their room every night, I will tuck my kids in. I would play the piano, sing or do something else to help them know that it was going to be OK. I needed to make sure their mindset was OK and that they knew we were going to make it. I had lost the use of most of the left side of my body. I couldn't feel anything from the waist down and I was using crutches. I remember telling Anna that when this was all over, we were going to do a 5K together (Anna loved runs). She said, you can't even walk, what are you talking about? I told her it that it didn't matter, we were going to do it. You just need to put it in your mind. I had her train for a whole year. At the very end of my treatment, when I was well enough to walk, I was able to walk the 5K. My best friend walked alongside me, as well as my mother in law. It was a very beautiful moment. I thought yes, we can get through this. We don't make it to everything. I'm not going to wave the victory flag, like everything is perfect in my life. However, I made it to this milestone. I'm going to celebrate it. We have some great pictures and my best friend even got me a medal to wear. I think when people realize the mindset, that is when you see the light switch click.

Naomi Damask

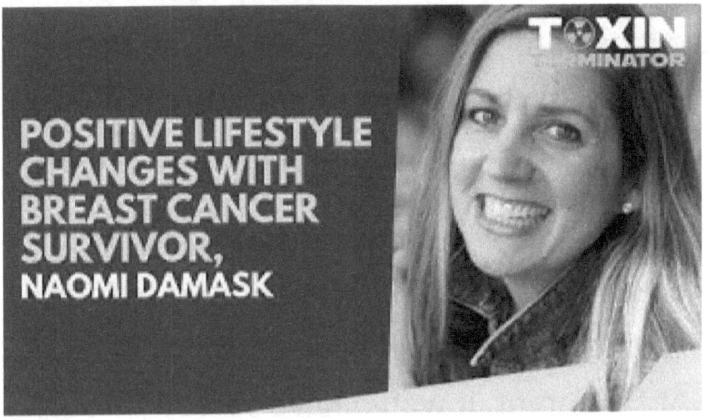

She is a breast cancer Thrivor. It was this diagnosis in December 2011 that set her on her passion of becoming a Wellness Warrior. Being diagnosed at such a young age, she really needed to take a look at why this was happening to her. She found out that less than 10% of cancer diagnoses are genetically related. That means over 90% have to do with our lifestyle choices. Naomi considers her cancer diagnosis a gift. Let's read her story of lifestyle change and stepping into your purpose.

 "I was diagnosed in December of 2011. People were saying, you are so young. Does it run in your family? People asked these questions all the time, because I was an athlete. I also seemed to be eating what I thought at the time to be clean. This journey, as a breast cancer survivor, has actually been a gift. I know people look at me cross eyed, when I say that. However, it has truly changed every area of my life. I am full of gratitude that I have a second chance.

I had two tumors when I was diagnosed. I felt one, but I didn't feel the other. This was actually a blessing because they said I would have probably been stage four. At that point, it would have spread throughout my entire body. I was under the age of 40, so mammograms were not on my radar. This is why self-breast exams are so important. I now educate people about health and wellness, especially on prevention and what we can be doing. I don't think people realize that there are many available tools that are not mainstream. However, we need to know about them, such as thermography. I am very passionate about prevention. It is possible to go down a rabbit hole. However, there is great information that is available. I tell people that it has been a lot of silver linings, because I've been able to help and give hope to many people who are recently diagnosed.

Our health and wellness have to do with our lifestyle and our environment. These are the biggest things. I am not just saying this. You can look at the research that has been done. There's a website called pubmed.gov, which is the National Institution of Health library, where you can find these research articles. There is a growing movement involving nutrigenomics and epigenetics. These are growing areas of sciences that demand your attention. People are getting sicker at an earlier age. However, we have so much more technology. It makes you wonder what is going on.

I feel like I overwhelm people when I discuss lifestyle and environmental changes. Sometimes I feel like they roll their eyes at me. I say to them that they are going to think that I am crazy, as I believe that our technology is part of the problem. The Wi-Fi is important, because it's disrupting our sleep. We go to bed and before we go to sleep, we are on our tablets and our phones. The blue light from these devices is disrupting our sleep cycles. It gives us a false sense of daylight and causes our hormones to get off balance. Some people are very sensitive to Wi-Fi, because of our genes. Everyone's genetic makeup is different, so this might not be a sensitivity for you. One of my daughters is extremely sensitive. When she is using her iPad, or her cell phone, she is a totally different child, compared to when she is out in nature. I tell people to stop wearing smart watches and Fitbits. They are emitting EMFs into our body. It is breaking down our cells. People need to realize that as much as we love the technology, we have to take a break from it. Our mind needs a break. Everyone thinks that wellness is about exercise and eating. However, we also need to rest our brains. We need to rest in meditation or prayer and just be quiet.

Our emotional and mental health is very important. There have been many studies, such as the one where they take two plants. They tell one plant I hate you, you're ugly. They then tell the other planet; you are beautiful, and you bring me love and joy. There is a notable difference in the growth and vitality of that plant. We are vibrations. We are energy, just like those plants. If we are full of hatred, think about what it is doing to the inside of you. It is very sad because many survivors have done everything from a holistic standpoint, but they were still full of fear and anger.

People also need to pay attention to what they are putting on their bodies. I used a deodorant that was clinically proven to help reduce sweat. When I look back at it now, it was going right into my lymph nodes, which is right in the breast area. Estrogen positive is the most common type of breast cancer. There are many things that mimic estrogen. The ingredients in deodorant have not only been to linked breast cancer, but also to Alzheimer's and dementia. I worked for Maybelline, where I learned that the ingredients that are allowed in the United States are very different than what is permitted in the European Union. They ban thousands of ingredients, while we only prohibit 20 ingredients. This is not restricted to personal care products. The same type of situation exists with major box corporations and the food sources. There are differences in the type of yogurt that is exported to the EU compared to what is sold here. Even the individual states vary in what they allow. There are products that get labeled differently in California than in New York.

When I received my diagnosis, I interviewed every single breast cancer survivor who would talk to me. I then did my homework. I knew that I wanted to do the all-natural approach. We lived in the City of Chicago at the time, which had many fantastic hospitals. However, I wanted to go to an alternative hospital. My husband completely disagreed with me. He said that I could green juice all I want afterwards. However, I had two little girls (a preschooler and a first grader). I negotiated with my husband because I did not want to do chemo.   I tell everyone that you must be your own advocate. It is your body and your mind, so you have to decide what you want to do. I ended up doing a bilateral mastectomy combined with chemo. However, I negotiated and only did four rounds. I was very blessed that my oncologist would work with me. In the cancer world, there are many differences of opinions regarding the appropriate treatment. It is my opinion that you must do what you think is best for you. I have no regrets. I don't live my life with regrets. I am happy. I made the best decision that I could make for myself. I am now continuing to build on that. If you do get diagnosed, even if you have a rock-solid marriage, you should go see a counselor together. You need to get the level of support you need for each other, because you will both need it.

I regularly do things now to help move my lymphatic system. The role of our lymphatic system is to remove the garbage from our bodies. It is one of our body's systems that is not linked to a major organ. This means that we must pump it manually to help move it through our body. Most people don't understand what the lymphatic system is. All they know is that if someone gets a cancer diagnosis, they say it was in their lymph nodes, which is bad. However, they don't understand anything else about it. It is actually linked to our immune system. One of the things that I do for my lymphatic system is dry brushing. Stimulating the lymphatic system using a dry brush is very important and it is something that we should do each day. I also talk about rebounding on mini trampolines, the up and down motion of rebounding on trampolines also pumps up the lymphatic system. Other techniques for stimulating the lymphatic system include hot cold showers and Crown cranial therapy. The Finnish people like to jump into freezing cold waters and then get into their saunas. The symptoms of the lymphatic system not working well are similar to what we see with toxin overload. The lymphatic system is responsible for garbage removal, which is similar to the role of the digestive system in the detox system. It involves moving everything out of the body.

I am totally blessed. I went on a personal growth journey. I asked God if he were to give me another chance, what would I do with it? I started to work on areas of my life that I could improve, like relationships. The key is to have healthy relationships and to set up boundaries. I choose not to be around people who are negative. I learned to say no. It did serve me well, because I was the room mom and was doing everything. My parties were amazing. As a result, I put a lot of extra stress upon myself. It is not worth it, I needed to learn to say no. I would advise you not to get overwhelmed and throw your hands up in the air. You need to remember the 80/20 rule. You don't have to be perfect.

Bobbi Schaben

My friend Bobbi Schaben is a homeschooling mom of four. This is a miracle, because at one time she was told that she would not be able to have children. She has such a beautiful story of knowing her body can heal and turning into her faith.

Like most people, I lived a regular life, eating and showering with all the junk and chemicals and thinking it was not going to hurt me. When I was 19, I noticed that my health started to go into a downward spiral. At that time, I was diagnosed with severely high blood pressure. It was so high that they got me into Mayo Clinic overnight. It usually takes months to get in. Over the next 11 years, I ended up having a whole bunch of things. I had severe pain in my plantar fasciitis and

Achilles tendonitis. It got to the point where I would crawl to the bathroom and sit on the counter to do the dishes. The pain was taking a toll. I was taking medication for the high blood pressure and then started on the painkillers. My immune system was very weak at the time. As a result, I was constantly taking antibiotics. They actually gave me a stash of antibiotics for my specific issues, with twelve refills. It was a complete downward spiral. I had very low energy and I was sick all the time. I thought that if it continued, I would be in a wheelchair by the time I was thirty-five. In 2002, I had my first Meniere's disease attack. It is a disease of your inner ear which is responsible for your body awareness and your balance. I would be perfectly fine, then all of a sudden with no warning I would lose my body awareness. During the first attack I couldn't turn on a light switch. Sometimes I wouldn't be able to walk, and I would vomit for hours. These attacks started happening every week and a half to two weeks or months. Since they were so unpredictable, it got to the point, that I lost my ability to drive. I was never diagnosed with anxiety, but I was afraid to go out. I didn't want to have an attack in public. I went to a hospital where they diagnosed me with Meniere's disease. I went to the Mayo Clinic, where they said I was too young, and didn't fit the usual profile. They said that I probably had benign positional vertigo. They conducted the Meniere's disease test. They usually put water in the ear, but at Mayo they used air since I had gotten very sick when they used water before. They said the air wasn't as intense. This triggers a Meniere's disease attack. I ended up on the floor in the doctor's office at the Mayo Clinic. The doctors were holding my hair back, as I threw up into the trash can. He said that he was wrong and that I did have Meniere's disease. He said that not only did I have it in one ear, I had it in both ears. This is pretty significant and pretty awful.

 My husband and I had been married for a few years and really wanted to have kids. However, we knew that I couldn't safely take care of a child. What if the child was crawling towards steps and I had an attack and I couldn't get to them? When we left the Mayo Clinic, they said I may get worse, but it won't get better. As you can imagine, when I left Mayo, I was at rock bottom. I am so thankful for my husband. He looked at me and said, Bobbi, God created you, don't you think he can heal you? I said, I have no doubt he can heal me. However, maybe he is using this and I'm willing. I didn't like to be willing, but I was. Instead of using it in my sickness, he would teach me how to get well, so that I could help others. We were at a point where the people of the world had given us no hope. Therefore, we turned to the Bible and followed those principles. In a matter of months, I was off of all my painkillers, blood pressure medicine and Meniere's disease medicines.

Our first discovery was Doctor Ted Broer's maximum health and fitness audio CD set. We started by realizing that we needed to treat my body like a temple. The Bible says that our bodies are a temple of the Holy Spirit. I would not walk into a church and bring in a bag of rotting garbage and just throw it all over. That is appalling, but it is what I had been doing to my body. It was necessary to remove the artificial colors, artificial flavors and all of those other horrible chemicals that are in our food. However, it was not only food, we also learned that anything that goes on our skin is actually being absorbed. Therefore, we were harming the temple when we put poisons on our skin. As a result, we really changed our diet. Many people want to do this one step at a time. However, I was very afraid of having another attack. It was the worst feeling in the world, so I was all in. We put a water filter on our shower heads and our drinking water at the time. We now have a filter for our entire house. I have learned that showering for 15 minutes in hot water is worse than drinking eight 8 oz glasses of contaminated water. This is because you are breathing in the steam. Your pores open up when it's hot and your skin absorbs like a sponge. We ate what they did in the Bible and did not eat what they didn't eat. We flushed out the toxins and fed our bodies the nutrients that it needed. I got results very quickly. As a result of the changes, I have not had a Meniere's disease attack since 2003.

I told somebody at church about the story. He told me, that he went home, did his research and found that it is not supposed to go away. He asked me if I meant to tell him that God just healed me. I told him that there are two kinds of healing in the Bible, laomai and therapeuo. Laomai is where He touches you or you are instantly healed. With therapeuo, He teaches you what you need to do and as you walk in obedience, you get well. Many of the healings in the Bible were therapeuo healings. He taught me what I needed to do. As I walked in obedience, my body was able to heal itself. I like to teach people what the Bible says about getting well. As they walk in obedience, they will also get results. I have always seen it work. We cannot plead the promises without practicing the principles. That is what I learned. God wants us to walk in divine health. If I wanted those results, then I needed to follow the principles.

I find that it is useful to present a visual, when discussing toxins. If you burned your hand, you would go to the doctor and use Aloe Vera or whatever the doctor gives you. However, if you don't take your hand off the stove, the burn will never go away. It, therefore, starts with taking your hand off. We have removed things like propylene glycol, which is in lotions. While there are warnings on paint cans about avoiding skin contact with propylene glycol, in lotions it is the second or third ingredient listed. It is also in salad dressings. We avoided products containing sodium laurel sulfate, phthalates and anything else that was artificial or synthetic. We stopped eating scavenger animals, which included shellfish and pork. As we were studying, we realized that you actually use more nutrition to digest these types of foods than you actually take in. There are different interpretations of what the New Testament says. You must decide whether or not it's healthy for you. When I made those changes I got better, despite everybody saying that I wouldn't. Although there are now many different fad diets, the Bible never changes. I have never seen it not work. We found that wheat was not bad. The einkorn only has 14 chromosomes. However, our wheat now has 43 chromosomes, and we wonder why we can't digest it, when it's been genetically modified. We are trying to get back to how they used to do it, which cannot be found in a grocery store. They used to rest the land during biblical time. However, that is usually not done anymore. When the soil is rested, it is replenished. The chemicals that are used deplete the vitamins from the soil. Since our soil doesn't have the nutrients that it used to, I take a whole food vitamin.

I don't think it is possible to completely avoid pesticides, since they are in the air. However, we always choose organic, especially for things with a thinner skin. If you are limited financially, it is most important to choose organic butter and milk. Even if the cows are grass fed, there are still pesticides in the grass. Since we store our toxins in our fat, the pesticides are going to be present in products with high fat content. This also applied to produce with thin skin like apples, strawberries and grapes. We focus on foods that help our body to detoxify, like cruciferous vegetables, such as cabbage and broccoli.

Essential oils are also very helpful, although I was skeptical at first. Essential oils are used in the Bible for health and wellness. I found that the oils supported our bodies in helping to clean up receptor sights and to nourish and detoxify our bodies. Since my background is in science, I found the science of essential oils to be very interesting. It explains why the various oils are used for the altar, protection and healing. It also helps us to understand why Jesus refused certain offerings on the cross but accepted others.

Our children assume that the things we give them are healthy. They will do what we do. Therefore, we should give them the precious gift of having the healthiest and purest environment possible. No matter what you are experiencing, it is a warning sign. It is a reminder that you need to change your ways and let your body heal itself. The truth is that not everyone has that opportunity. They have conditions that appear suddenly and take them down very fast.

Melissa Rupp

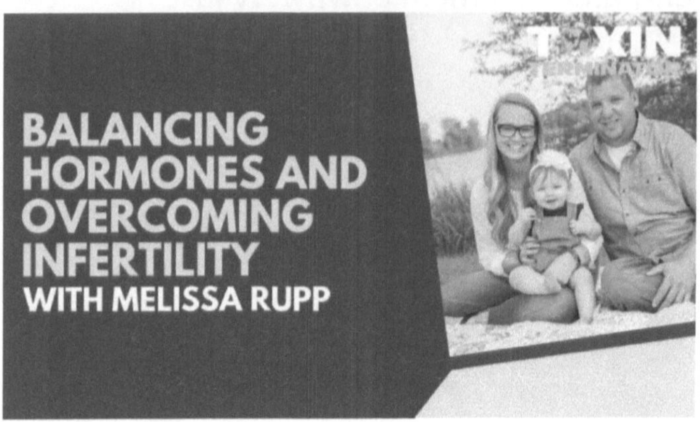

I met Dr. Melissa Rupp, a chiropractor in northwest Iowa, through my daughter-in- law. She has always been in tune to learning how the body worked and choosing more natural modalities to get to the root of any issue. She has an incredible story to share about her very personal journey of infertility. She has now added women's services into her chiropractic office.

"My story actually started when I was 12 years old. We think that when we are teenagers our female system is just kind of a mess. In reality, it is but I guess I always just felt like mine was a bigger mess than everybody else's. It's one of those things that you don't really think too much about, until you get older, get married and start to talk about having kids. When things aren't quite happening the way they're supposed to and your cycle is a mess, is when you start to look back. You realize, hey wait a minute, this all started when I was 12 years old. It didn't wait until I was 30. This has been happening for years. You start to put those little pieces together. I am someone who really likes to educate myself. I like to understand the science behind why my body does what it does and what I need to do to make it work better. It was a big educational time when all of this happened, to be able to look back at my life and figure out that this is why I am like this and what I should have done. It's one of those times in life, where you wish you knew then what you know now. This experience has really changed my perspective on what women's health should be. It made me angry that I didn't know the things I should have known and that my mom didn't know. My mom took her 12-year-old daughter, who had a period for two straight months, to see the doctor. I was missing school. My period was so incredibly heavy, that I was anemic. I was in so much pain that I couldn't get off the floor. I was living on ibuprofen and Tylenol and other painkillers, and I was only 12 years old. As a mom, I look back at what my mom had to go through in dealing with me and having absolutely no idea what to do. The first thing that the doctor said was, "we'll put her on the pill and that will take care of it. If we put her on birth control, it will fix all of her problems, regulate the cycle and she'll be all normal. Everything will be perfect".

If you don't know how the birth control pill works, you need to do some research. It has a major internal effect on your hormones. It is the main reason why we ended up on the infertility journey. I hadn't even had my period for a year, before I was put on the pill. I took it starting when I was 12 years old, until I went off it when I was about 30. It seems normal for women to be put on birth control pills. It is just what they do. Most women think that the pill regulates the period. However, did you know that when you are on the pill, you don't actually get a period? It is not your period; it is breakthrough bleeding. The pill was designed to make you feel like you are still getting a period, so you can still "feel normal". I don't think that there is anything natural about it. We have taken those hormones for many years upon years for women. It is a special problem for younger girls who are trying to figure out what their bodies are doing. They start taking hormones to regulate themselves and it just shuts them down. The birth control movement started in the early 1900s, in response to a concern for childbirth and the fear of self-induced abortions for low-income women. During World War 1, servicemen being treated for venereal diseases. Women at this time were under the impression that having a baby and dealing with your period, were going to keep them from being able to support themselves or their family, while their husband was at war. We have, therefore, developed the mentality that everything that makes us a woman, will let us down and hold us back. This is entirely untrue!

We started this journey many years ago but didn't realize it. When we got married, I went off the pill. We decided to try, but not really try to get pregnant. After about a year and a half, we decided that we were ready and really wanted to get pregnant. We were 30 when we got married, so we wanted to settle down and have a family. When it started to become difficult, I began to do my own research using charting. As a result, I learned how hormone levels work and that when they change, your body temperature changes. When you are early in your cycle, your temperature will tend to stay somewhat lower. Following ovulation, your body temperature would rise significantly and then fall again right around menstruation. I began doing this charting and noticed that my chart wasn't looking like it should. During this time, my cycle had gotten very abnormal. I ended up having a period that was extremely scary. I got really sick at work.   I somehow got home but I have no recollection of how I did it. My husband returned home about four hours after I did. While I was sitting in the chair, I was very pale and didn't feel like I was there. I was bleeding very heavily and throwing up, I also had a terrible headache and my ears were ringing. I never felt so horrible in my life. This was not long after going off the pill. My husband looked at me and he was scared because he didn't know if I was OK. That was the awakening moment for us.

During my research I found a doctor who I had seen before. She felt that it is more of a fertility issue, since we were thinking about getting pregnant. She, therefore, recommended a fertility doctor. The fertility doctor told us that our two options were get pregnant or go on the pill. Neither of these two solutions sounded good to us. This is another hindsight is 2020 moments. I like to share my story because I encounter many women in my office who have had similar experiences. We worked with the fertility doctor for a while. He was willing to help us have a baby, which is what we were trying to do. The doctor had me do some different charting. When he looked at my charts, he said that according to my temperatures, I was not ovulating. He told us I had what is called an anovulatory cycle. With this type of cycle, you don't ovulate, but you bleed. I had never heard of this type of cycle before. I don't necessarily believe it, because I was having some serious menstrual bleeding and pain. In this charting, I was taking my temperature every single morning. I was then putting it on a chart and watching it. Your charting will show you when you ovulate. This made me think that the time you are ovulating, you should have intercourse if you want to get pregnant. Your temperature rises, then falls, and it will spike. When it spikes, it means your progesterone is high, which occurs after you ovulate. It is the hormone that helps build up your endometrium to accept a fertilized egg for implantation, so you can get pregnant and stay pregnant. Progesterone is a very good warming hormone. It is why your temperature gets higher during the second half of your cycle. As your estrogen falls, your progesterone rises. They work in sync with each other. My chart went up and then it didn't fall. It would stay level and then rise.

 Based on this information, he told me that I wasn't ovulating. He put me on several different medications, including clomid. Three months later, he put me on a different medication. Clomid has some significant effects on your body. It actually causes you to ovulate. However, it can also cause hyper-ovulation. In this situation, you ovulate more eggs than you should. As a result, your ovaries get overwhelmed. It can cause tremendous weight gain. I gained 10 pounds during the three months that I was on it. In the fourth month, it bumped me up into a new BMI where I was considered to be overweight. I, therefore, had to take a different pill, since I was now overweight. However, it was caused by the clomid they put me on in the first place. This gives you an idea of what these medications can do. It also made me feel like a crazy person. I remember wondering why my husband would want to have a baby with me, when I don't even like myself. I was angry, crabby, losing my hair, gaining weight and my skin was like I was 12 years old again. I was an absolute mess and it was because of all the medications I was taking. It made me wonder if this is what we need to do in order to have the one thing in the world that I want, which is a baby? It was insane! That was when we both decided that we needed to figure something else out. We felt something else going on, and this approach was not treating what was causing it. The doctor wasn't paying attention to my symptoms, heavy periods and abnormal cycles. He didn't care, because his only goal was to get you pregnant. We agreed that we couldn't do this anymore. It would lead to a divorce, if we stayed on this present course. It was making us too unhappy in both our marriage and our lives.

At this point, I started the journey of figuring out how these things have affected my life, my body and my hormones and what could I do to fix it. I always believed that I had endometriosis, because the symptoms were always there. Those symptoms include constipation, bloating and diarrhea with your cycle. It is around the time of your actual period. Some people have pain with intercourse, bowel movements, and urination, painful cycles, mood swings, acne, weight gain or difficulty losing weight. It is also common to have abnormal cycles (some are heavy while others are not). The length of the periods can also vary. The most serious symptom I had was very intense pain with my period. I had pap smears every year, since I was twelve years old. I would also talk to my doctor all the time. I use five different types of birth control over the years. Every few years my "period" (remember it isn't actually your period) would get very bad again and the cramps would be very strong. I would then tell the doctor that it wasn't helping. They would then put me on a different type of birth control pill. However, every time I mentioned endometriosis, they would say that I didn't have it or if I did, the pill would cure it. When you are young, you don't really understand everything. Therefore, you take their word for it. There are many doctors who truly care. They are much more holistic. One doctor who I admire tells me to listen to your inner voice. If your mind is telling you that they're not telling you the truth, you need to find a different doctor.

Through my research, I have learned that an endometriosis diagnosis requires a laparoscopic study. It' is the type of surgery where they make an incision in your abdomen, and then use an internal camera to examine and diagnose certain diseases that you cannot be seem on an ultrasound, CT or MRI. This type of procedure is not done by every doctor. It is not something that they will do, unless they feel like they have to. I didn't really push it. However, I knew that endometriosis is an inflammatory disease. There is an endometrial lining on the inside of your uterus. Following ovulation, progesterone allows the endometrium to become thick. Therefore, when a fertilized egg comes down, it will be able to implant. If it's not fertilized, it sloughs off and you get your period. With endometriosis, there are clumps of endometrial cells that grow on the outside of the uterus. They are growing inside of your abdomen. In some women, it attaches to their bowels. Other women have adhesions that will attach your ovary to your uterus or to your bowel. Those are very severe cases. With endometriosis, it doesn't matter how bad it is, because it has no effect on your symptoms. Some women have large lesions, but they don't have any real symptoms. By contrast, other women (like me) with mild cases, have severe symptoms. These cells act the same way outside the uterus, as they do inside of it. When they are attached to your colon or the internal parts of your body, they grow, inflame and slough off. This causes a buildup of excess blood inside areas of your abdomen, which results in more inflammation. The reason why endometriosis causes the pain, is due to the inflammatory part that people don't always understand.

Since I now understood this, I had to identify possible changes with my diet that would help me to reduce the inflammation. I had learned about thyroid function in school. I also thought that there might be a problem with my thyroid. I had always worked out a lot and was very athletic. However, I was always on the heavier side. I wasn't overweight, but I wasn't as lean as I should with all the exercising that I had done. I was never a runner, but I liked to lift. I liked to do things that helped to build lean muscle mass, which allows you to lose fat faster. I found out that the thyroid dysfunction caused excess weight gain which is very difficult to lose. It also caused other symptoms like brittle hair and skin issues. I had those symptoms as well as eczema and acne. I started to eat healthier. I was also using essential oils to help my body to be able to detox and to be able to mentally get used to the major changes that I was going to need to make. I started eating a lot of fruits, vegetables and eliminated dairy and wheat. I started to take supplements and use essential oils that were aimed to support my thyroid. I knew that would help my body to take care of itself. I wasn't diagnosed with anything. I just wanted to make sure my thyroid was working the way that it should.

In three months, I had lost weight, which I hadn't been able to do in years. I had lost 10 pounds and I was feeling really good. I was still doing my charting and tracking. At this point, we were not trying to get pregnant. We just said that we needed a break. We found out that we were pregnant. My charting was the same as always and we are pregnant. I thought that it was crazy, because I was told that I don't ovulate. I went to the doctor, who did an ultrasound and said that I was pregnant. They thought that I was about six weeks and should come back at eight weeks. I stopped taking one of the supplements, because it had increased the amounts of iodine. However, I was still doing all the other things. I then started spotting, which made me really nervous. The spotting continued. I went in to get checked out and we ended up having a miscarriage. To this day, my husband swears that it was because of my thyroid, since I stopped taking the supplement for my thyroid. I changed how I looked at it because of additional knowledge. However, I think that did it play a big part in it. It was also the endometriosis and finding out many things about my hormones. I feel like there have been many times over those years where things were enlightening for me. Then all of a sudden, there was a new enlightenment.

We sat in the doctor's office. Between my tears, he was very blunt and almost rude to us. I think that doctors see so many miscarriages that they get numb to them. He told us our next option was to see a reproductive endocrinologist, who would look at IVF. This was something that we were not morally ready to do. We weren't ready to take this step yet. I didn't know if we were ever going to be ready for it. The other option was clomid. I was asking why because we already tried that. The doctor had told me we couldn't get pregnant, because I don't ovulate (but I did). He told us it must have been a fluke. It was so appalling, that we walked out of his office very deflated. My husband is a very quiet man, who doesn't say much. However, he looked at me and said, "we're never going back there, never again." He may have said a few other words. This was really a turning point in our marriage. Sometimes you have to go through horrible things for you to wake up and realize what you have and what you're working towards. I asked my doctor what causes miscarriage. He said that we don't know. I asked if I could be tested. He said that they don't do it until after three times. I said you're telling me I have to lose three babies, before you're going to even care. The most upsetting part to John, was the doctor's blatant, oh well attitude.

After the miscarriage, I had taken a week for myself. I decided I needed some time for self- reflection and time to mourn. We both were at the point where we knew there had to be something better. I wanted answers why my body wasn't doing, what it is meant to do. There was something wrong with it and we needed to be able to fix it. We both said that no matter what, we need to heal me. If we can't have children, we can't have children. That was beside the point. I needed to heal, because he remembered the really bad period. He thought that I was 30 years old and I couldn't live like that until I was 50 or 60. That was not OK. I, therefore, decided to do more research. I looked at the different doctors in our area. I also looked randomly at all the different hospitals. I wanted to see who was there, what they had to offer and whether there was anybody, anywhere that people would recommend. I came across a doctor by the name of Dr. Harrison Hanson. I looked at a picture of him and two women. At the bottom, it said, "Orange City Fertility Care Center" (now Ashwood Fertility Care Center). It piqued my curiosity, because I was under the impression the only place that did anything with fertility was Sioux Falls or Sioux City. We live in northwest Iowa and there's just nothing here. It is an hour and a half drive each way to get to somewhere that does this. I started looking into it and I fell in love with everything that they had to offer. Orange City

Fertility Care Center teaches a method of natural family planning. They use charting that is actually taught to you, instead of taking your temperature every day. They are able to look at your chart and determine if there are any underlying issues related to your fertility. They then refer you on to a doctor, who looks at your chart. He says that based on your charting, this is what we see.   They teach the Creighton Model Fertility Care System. With this system, you do not chart your temps, ovulation sticks, symptoms, etc., you chart your cervical mucus. After I found this program, I showed it to John. We liked that they stated, "to treat underlying issues to enhance your fertility and enhance the likelihood of becoming pregnant". This was exactly what we were looking for. We wanted to find out what was going on, so that we could treat those things. I truly believed that if I could treat those things, I could get pregnant.

The first step was to do what I could at home. We knew that my hormones were a disaster. Therefore, we had to remove the things that disrupted them. This included sulfates, parabens, phthalates, and artificial colors and dyes. We found these items in our hair products, face products, soaps and foods. THEY WERE IN EVERYTHING. I was suddenly reading every single label that I saw. This was because every single product that I used had five to 25 ingredients that were disrupting my hormones. It made me realize that we needed to clean up our bodies. The effects of these toxins begin to affect us as children without our knowledge. By the time that we become adults, we feel terrible. It takes time for our bodies to realize what they are supposed to do, what they are meant to do, and they must do to get rid of all that excess clutter. The next step was to begin our Creighton Model Charting. We went to the introductory session without a practitioner. We were shocked at the large volume of information about my body and fertility that we weren't aware of. We began charting and had frequent follow-up appointments with our practitioner to make sure that we understood what we were looking for and what we were seeing. After seeing two cycles of charting, we were referred to a physician.

We met with Dr. Hanson, who looked at our chart that I had been doing for two months. He said that I had endometriosis, polycystic ovarian syndrome, a thyroid dysfunction, low progesterone and possibly a uterine infection. He could tell almost all of that just by looking at what my cervical mucus did for a month. That was it. He had recommendations for diet and other things, many of which I was already doing. However, he also referred me to Dr. Pakiz at the Saint Paul VI Institute for Reproductive Health in Omaha, Nebraska. He informed me that I needed to have a

surgical consult for my endometriosis. Saint Paul VI
Institute in Omaha is the reproductive health clinic that
developed the Creighton Model and NaPro technology.
Natural procreative technology diagnoses and treats
underlying issues to help enhance fertility. One of the
things that people ask me all the time, is how do you
get your health insurance to pay for fertility
treatment? Most insurance plans don't allow payment
for infertility as a diagnosis. NaPro Technology
considers infertility to be a secondary condition, that is
caused by many other primary conditions. In my case,
it was endometriosis, PCOS, underactive thyroid, and
low progesterone. They believe if they can treat those
underlying conditions, then infertility often does not
exist. In some individuals, infertility is legitimate.
However, for most people these conditions can be
treated, which will allow them to have babies
naturally. That is what they sent me down there for.
After six months, we had laparoscopic surgery where
they actually excised my endometriosis. It isn't just a
laser where they burn it off, they literally cut it out
completely. This decreases the risk of the
endometriosis returning. There are only a few places
that do this surgery, so we waited six months. During
that period, they gave us other things to do. I went on
an anti-inflammatory diet, which required me to cut
out dairy, soy, gluten and sugar. They had me do
progesterone tests every two weeks, which required

blood draws. I had to have the levels drawn daily for two weeks post-ovulation, so that they could actually see where my progesterone levels were, in relation to a normal healthy post- ovulation cycle. Charting my cervical mucus was very interesting. It made us realize that I wasn't ovulating, when my temperatures should show that I was. I was actually ovulating about eight days later, which explains how we became pregnant! It is very interesting because I learned many things about my body. This included that your cycle can show you when you are sick or stressed. Your cervical mucus can show you the changes in your body.

After six months, and it was finally time for my surgery. My surgery took almost four hours, although they assumed it would take only two. They kept John informed the entire time about what they were doing and finding. Dr. Pakiz was amazing! She said that my case was mild to moderate. However, instead of coming back for another robotic surgery to remove the larger lesions, she decided to do them now. I was able to go home the next day and returned three days later for my follow-up. She showed me parts of the surgery on video, which I got to keep. I saw what my polycystic ovary looked like. She also removed a few tubal cysts, that were weighing down my fallopian tubes. I also saw where she was able to remove the endometriosis from different areas in my abdomen. It was surreal to finally feel that someone heard me. I realized that something I felt for years was real and was now gone. Following the surgery, they performed an ultrasound series to actually view my ovaries and determined that they were actually ovulating. I went every single day for 13 days for internal ultrasounds. They started me on compounded, bioidentical progesterone. I take progesterone pills for 10 days out of every month. They also started me on a thyroid regimen. I dropped 12 pounds and I had never felt better. My hair quit falling out, my eczema went away, and my skin got better. At the same time, I was using very good supplements and good body care products. All of these steps together, really helped us. I had my first normal cycle in 15 to 20 years in November. In December, we were pregnant and went on to have our beautiful rainbow baby, Willa, in September 2017.

The biggest takeaway that I hope women have gotten from our journey, is to be aware of what your body is made to do. Women were not meant to have abnormal or painful periods. We were meant to ovulate, menstruate and gestate. We were given this amazing ability. Shutting that down with hormones, will not help you hormonally. It will only delay the inevitable. If you take the pill to "fix" your female problems and then one day you decide to stop taking it, those underlying conditions are still going to be there. The pill WILL NOT CURE anything. I want women to know that there are other available options. They do not undermine your feminine being. The Creighton Model is a system that works for women in all stages in life. This includes: if you want to have a baby, are peri menopausal, or if you don't want to have children but you want to know what's going on in your body. It can even be helpful for preteens. It can tell you many things about your body and it is for everybody. It is not just for getting pregnant. After the birth of our daughter, I decided that this system changed our lives for the better. More women deserve to know how their bodies work. I also wanted to be able to help other women who felt lost and frustrated with their infertility journeys. I decided to start training with the Saint Paul VI Institute. I am currently working with Ashwood Fertility Care Center in Orange City, Iowa. We have some great practitioners at the center. We see clients in person, as well as online from anywhere. If you are looking for a more natural way to be able to plan your family or want help with your cycles/fertility, I would love to help! I wish all women could understand and respect the great abilities that our bodies have been given, because they truly are a blessing!

Melissa Rupp DC, FCPI

Sarah Steele

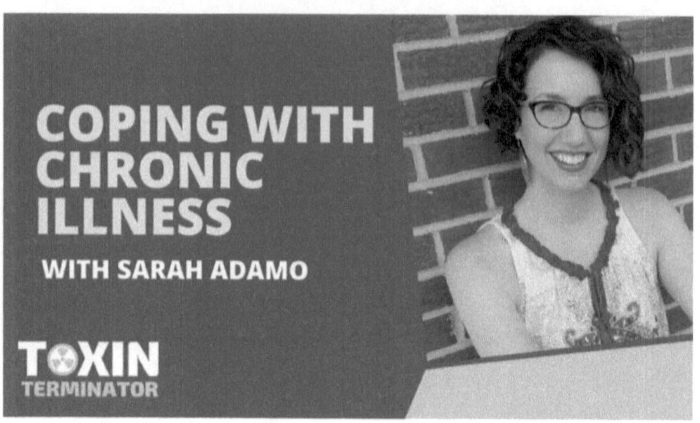

My friend Sarah Steele will share her story that originally started as a teenager, when she got the first two series of the hepatitis B vaccination, which ended up injuring her. This injury caused her to try to heal her body through the conventional medical route. However, she found that she wasn't getting any relief. Therefore, she started to learn about the concept of toxins in her environment and inside her home. She found what she was eating was making a difference in her overall health. Not only was she trying to improve her own health, but as a mother of seven (and now 10) she was empowering her children. She didn't want to have them share her story.

"My story began in the 1990s, when the vaccine schedule was limited starting at birth and the hep B vaccine was new to the scene and was strongly promoted in high schools. There was literature sent out to all the students on the benefits of having the hepatitis B vaccine and the dangers of college situations. The literature did not mention that it was a STD (Sexually Transmitted Disease). Otherwise, I would have probably thrown it away. I intended to save myself for marriage, which I did. Therefore, I believed the propaganda on the paper and I got the first round of three injections. I had a reaction to the injection, so I went to the nurse and explained my situation. She told me I got the shot in one arm and I had the reactions in both arms, so it could not be from the shot. Doing my research later, I found that this was total baloney.   I had hard-painful lumps develop in both arms. They were primarily on the back of each arm in the fatty tissue. They were hot to the touch and very painful. These lumps were very close to the injection site and developed within a few days. This has never happened before. I knew it wasn't a muscle issue. It was definitely a hard and painful lump. I was trying to figure out what was going on. Because it was dismissed as not being related to the vaccine, it was not reported as an adverse reaction. What most people don't understand is that even something as small as a fever, is still considered an adverse reaction. How many kids have fevers after receiving their immunizations? The nurse had me take a painkiller and then get my second round of the three-part series. I was dumb enough to believe her and I had the second round. With the second round of injections, I got the same kind of lumps in my arms and also in my legs. At this time, my parents decided that I was not going to get a third round. They wanted to figure out what this was and how to get rid of it. We spent the next six months going from specialist to specialist. At one point, I was told if the next test comes back positive, there is a chance that you may have less than six months to live. I was only 16 at the time. I was thinking that my life was coming to an end soon. I continued having biopsies, until they finally came up with a diagnosis. We tried many different drugs to see what would help. I was finally put on Prednisone, with some intermittent steroids in between to help with the pain. The Prednisone never made it go away. However, for important events like the prom, you take the steroids because without them you can't move. The problem was that whenever I took the steroids, the pain would come back worse than it was before. I always had to weigh my options. Was it really worth it to be pain free for one night, when I knew that the lumps and the pain would come back even worse than before?

We found out that the lumps were a hardening of the subcutaneous fatty layer of my skin between the skin and the muscle. Whenever there was pressure on that lump, either pressure from the underneath of the muscle moving or outside pressure from tight clothing or a chair or even sitting or lying in bed it was extremely painful. If you touched them with your finger, tears would just well up in my eyes. Walking and lying down became very painful.   I was seen by a dermatologist every month. They would take my blood to check for liver failure due to the Prednisone. Every six months they would check to make sure I wasn't going blind from the drugs. When I look back at that time, I ask what was I doing to myself? It is a very good thing that I didn't drink, because I was already ruining my liver with the Prednisone. However, I was at a point in my life, where the doctors know best. You trust what they're telling you to do. You don't know that there are other ways to treat yourself.

I finally did get a diagnosis. It is called chronic erythema nodosa. Erythema just means hot and red and nodosa are nodules under the skin. It is, therefore, just a description of what I had. The most common cause is birth control, although I had never been on birth control. I tried every drug listed for this condition with no luck, so we just ended up sticking with the Prednisone.   At this time, I was finishing high school, entering college and I had just gotten engaged. Three months after we were married, I found out that I was pregnant with my first child. I called up my dermatologist to inquire about the Prednisone. I knew that Prednisone stops rapidly dividing cells, like a baby. He told me to definitely wean myself off of it. This should be a warning that says you shouldn't take this drug if you're pregnant or nursing. There are also all of the blood tests checking for liver failure and blindness. While I was pregnant, I was thinking that I can't take these drugs, now what? I didn't know what to do. The standard American diet was how I was raised. We were not earthy, crunchy or organic by any means. In fact, we rarely had fresh fruits and vegetables at my house.

Most of those things came from a can. My mom did the best she could with what she had. She was a great mom but that's just how we were raised. The most important thing to remember in all of this, is baby steps and grace. I think so many people look at me and think that I've been doing organic all my life. However, I have not. I had Papa John's pizza 13 days straight, when I was pregnant. That is what I was craving. I didn't know that it was probably calcium that I needed instead of pizza, but pizza tasted good.

I just kind of lived through the pain during the pregnancy. I didn't think there was any alternative. I knew there had to be things that I could do to help naturally, and I needed to start looking into it. I looked into Doctor Mercola. He was going through a series on removing toxins from your home and detoxing your home. I thought, I have toxins in my home, so let's remove them. We started with the frying pans and we got rid of Teflon. I learned about my plastic shower curtain. When plastics are heated, they release toxins into the air. Therefore, we replaced the plastic shower curtain and threw away all our plastic kitchen containers. My husband saw that I was having a blast and seemed happy, so he was onboard. There are so many times that our husbands and our family think we're absolutely crazy. I did get labeled a little crazy. However, he felt that as long as I wasn't affecting his lifestyle too much, he was good. I started going down the rabbit hole. The thing that I notice the most is when I look at pictures of myself when I was pregnant with my first baby. I knew nothing about nutrition and toxins and all that stuff. I used all the scented stuff. I used everything and I gained 50 pounds, while I was pregnant. The majority of the weight was in my neck, my arms and my legs. I had a very small baby. However, small for me was 7 pounds, 6 ounces. Labor was hard and I had to have stitches after he was born. It was just not a good first pregnancy.

We found out we were pregnant for the second time. The second time around I had started learning about nutrition through The Weston A. Price Foundation. We started looking into raw milk, whole grains and other things that I had never heard about before. I ate very differently the second time around. However, I still gained 50 pounds. This time the 50 pounds were in my belly. My face looked about the same as when I was not pregnant, and my arms were the same. Most of it was all belly and the baby. Our second child was 10 pounds, five ounces. I've had bigger babies than that. Bigger babies are easier to deliver than smaller babies. You shouldn't worry about the size of your baby. Your body can handle it. We all know what contractions are. They are your uterus shrinking down. If you have a big baby, it has less to shrink down to get to the baby, than if you have a small baby. Therefore, you have fewer contractions to get to the baby and start pushing the baby out. You get quicker results. When you' are eating healthy and when you're consuming good quality products, you have good skin elasticity, very important for when you want to have a big baby. The second time, our baby was amazingly healthy. One of the nurses held him and told us you didn't see babies like this anymore. He had so much brown fat, he could not eat for three days and be fine. I think that was my first real world experience with what you eat really does matter. When you can see a baby and the differences in your labor and delivery, you realize how much nutrition matters. We are what we eat.

When you think about it, everything that your body makes has to come from what you eat and the air you breathe. If you're not breathing clean air and eating good food, you're giving your body very basic things to build itself with yet expecting the same results. You are just not going to get it. When I realized this, we started making little changes over time. This was when I had to bring my husband on board. I shared what I was learning and why I was so excited about it. I asked if he was willing to make these changes with me, for our family. He was totally on board, as long as I didn't start cutting out all of his favorite foods. We did have to switch him from the Kraft macaroni to homemade macaroni. There was a little bit of now you're really encroaching here. However, I just had him try it for a little while, since it was his favorite food. He did try it. However, for his birthday, he wanted to go back and have a box of Kraft. I told him to go for it. I said that you needed to have some freedom sometimes. After he ate it, he came back and was very disappointed. He told me that I ruined it for him. You really have to find what works for you. I think some people think when we talk about getting healthy, you have to cut out all this stuff. You might not, and others might. You have to do what is right for you. Everybody's got to have that mindfulness. When was the last time that you felt your body? It means that you really sat in the presence of your body and felt what it was doing.

I went through a kind of health transformation. It is now 2017. It has been 20 years since the vaccine. However, I was still in a lot of pain. It was not as much as before, but it was just something that I learned to live with. I had reduced it quite a bit. I had cleaned up our home. There were not as many changes as I would have liked. However, I still saw some. This has been going on for 20 years. I might do this gluten and dairy free thing. However, this scared me because so many changes are required. However, there are now many other options, which I appreciate. In full disclosure, if you're going to go dairy free, you are going to be depressed for a couple days. It is totally normal. You will dream of ice cream. I used to sit and think I missed that feeling in my mouth of melted cheese and ice cream. However, I also realized that it might not be forever. The way I would feel afterwards, would be worth it. Cutting out gluten and most dairy, reduced my pain by 80%. If I had the slightest bit of dairy, within 15 minutes, the pain would come back. I was so disappointed. Why did it have to be dairy? I've had friends who had gluten and dairy allergies who go to Europe and they can eat gluten and dairy. They have no problems with it. That got me going down the toxin trail. What is being put in our food here in the United States that's not being used in Europe? I started digging into GMO's. We were gluten free, no dairy and now no GMO's.

 People look at you and think that you are one of those health nuts. I love to share my story. It wasn't that I just couldn't wait to get rid of dairy in my diet. That was not it at all. I wasn't trying to be holier than thou. I just know that for my body and for me, it was a no. You sit there and enjoy your cheesecake. I am going to clap for you. I will also probably wish that I was you for about five minutes. However, I'm not having any, because it's not worth it to me. I know how I feel without it and I feel better. Until I heal my gut, which I truly believe will happen since God's going to do the healing, I'm going to put in the building blocks that my body needs to fix itself. God is going to work his magic in there. I have to figure out what building blocks I am missing in my body, so my body can do its job. God made us in a way, so that we fix ourselves. If you cut your finger, you don't have to put stuff on it to heal. You should wash it to get the germs out. However, your body is going to fix it all by itself. You don't even have to think about it. However, you have to put the things in your body to be able to fix it.

I also started cutting out all of the toxins from our environment. I learned that laundry detergent affects your reproductive system and putting dryer sheets in with your undergarments   puts toxins next to your reproductive system all day long. You are also sleeping in it and you are wrapping yourself up in it, after you get out of the shower. I don't want that for my children. I have my own story, but it doesn't have to be my kids' story. When they were growing up, our goal was to make sure that my children grew up in the cleanest possible environment.   This means that I tried to make it as toxin free as possible. This meant that it stopped at my door. I will not have fragrance in my home, and I won't have chemicals in my laundry detergent because my kids' lives matter. Because of what I've had to go through, I would never want them to go through that. If I have a chronic illness for the rest of my life, it was my choice to get the shot. However, my kids don't have to live out those poor choices. I want them to know better from the start. I teach them about nutrition. This empowers them to know what drinking a soda does to your body. You do control what's happening within the four walls of your home. You can't control what happens outside of it. The bottom line is that I want better for my kids. What convinced me this was the right way to raise your children, is when I heard someone say that your children will learn about God, by watching you as their parent. If you do not act as the authority in their life and teach them to submit to an authority from an early age as their parent, then how are they going to submit to the authority of God who they can't see? When I heard that, I thought it was a lot of responsibility. Parenting is a big responsibility. When you have seven children you can't make multiple dinners. If they don't eat the dinner, they won't starve themselves and eventually they will eat what you put in front of them. How you deal with that, is totally up to you as a parent. I keep explaining to them that I do it because I love them. I want what is best for their growing body. Since I know more about your body and nutrition than you do, you are going to listen to me.

I like to say that every choice has a consequence. If you decide to smoke cigarettes, eventually you will see the signs of aging from smoking earlier, than you would if you didn't smoke cigarettes. Every choice has its consequences. That includes our food, our willingness to exercise or to go outside in the sunshine. All of these things have potential consequences (both good and bad). Therefore, knowing that you have a choice, what are you going to choose? If you could look at yourself in the future, when you're retired, when you're in a nursing home, what do you want to look like? I look at women in their 80s who are up walking around and hanging out with their friends. I think that's who I want to be when I grow up. I want to be out living life and not crippled or incapacitated by my choices in life. I think that if you have that image, you work back from there. You can make good healthy choices, one at a time You don't have to go into your pantry and throw everything out. I was tempted to do that. However, you first have to realize that you have a choice. I think many of us walk around doing things, because that is how we have always done them. We don't realize that we can do better. However, we first had to know better, before we could do better. Just because you don't know something, don't beat yourself up about it. You can't undo the knowledge in your head, once you have it. That is true in many different areas of our life. If you go out and make poor decisions after you have the knowledge in your head, it is not as fun nor as enjoyable. This is because you know it isn't the best choice. It doesn't mean being healthy is the opposite of fun. You can still have fun.

I am now very passionate about letting people know that there is education out there for them, so they can make educated decisions for themselves. It is not one size fits all. You need to learn about your body and how you work. This will enable you to make the best choices for you and your children.

Donna Haugen

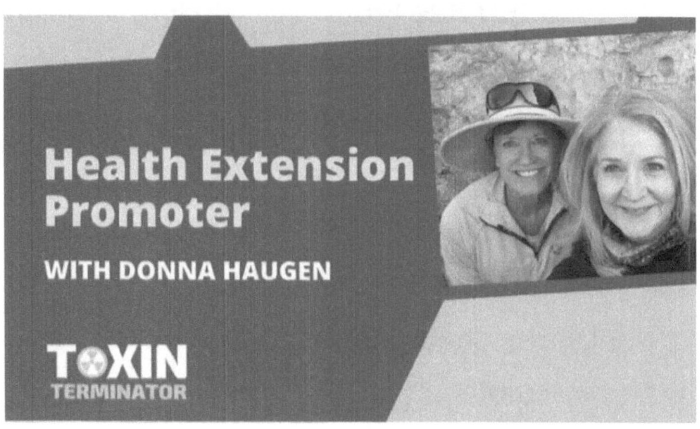

My final story to share is one from a very recent friend of mine, who has overcome breast cancer that had metastasized to her spine. I call her the "Queen of Biohacking", because this is how she not only survived, but thrived. At sixty years old, she now has the cells of a young thirty-year-old.

"I think my mother owns the original Prevention magazine. She was milking the goats and feeding the milk to the babies. Therefore, natural ways of living have always been a part of my life. I started my deeper dive when my daughter was two and got a constant runny nose. I didn't think that this was normal. I knew that something was causing it. I took her to an allergist, who used a computer and trigger points. It was all about energy and wavelength showing up on the computer to determine what was causing the reaction in my daughter. From his test, I cleaned out every toxin in my house. This included every chemical, perfume and the deodorant. We cleaned with just vinegar. Of course, we took her off of milk, wheat and sugar. We also did a rotation diet. He also made up drops for her. In two weeks, the child did not have a runny nose. It truly was miraculous. It all works.

Removing toxins and letting our bodies heal naturally is not new. It is now becoming more prevalent. We're shouting it from the rooftops, because of all the illness. People are getting ill faster and people are having reactions to all the things that they were exposed to on a daily basis. This leads right into the biohacking, because a lot of the exposures we can't get away from. We can't get away from EMF, our cell phones, computers, lights and everything else that we are exposed to on a daily basis. We can't just run away and live in the forest. Therefore, the most important thing is to recognize that. Don't be afraid, acknowledge that, then ask how to do I get my body back to homeostasis? I've attacked it all day long by just living my life. Now I need tools to combat that, because your body is miraculous. It can heal itself, if you put it in the proper environment. For instance, your sleep sanctuary. That is a perfect place to keep clean and peaceful and take out the EMF's, electricity and your cell phone out of there. You also need to get the lights out of there and let your body heal.

Even though you might know what is right and wrong, what to eat, how to exercise, the best lifestyle to live, we still don't always make the right choice. At about 55 years of age, I was living the life. I truly was superwoman. I was on top of the world and everything was going great. The next thing you know, I was being treated for breast cancer and it was shocking. I think part of my journey, is that you accept the messy with the beautiful and you recognize that there is no perfection. On the one hand, I did many things right. However, on the other side, I did things that I knew were potentially harmful to me. I never really investigated why I got the cancer diagnosis. It was just one of those things. If you're sick, you're sick and you get fixed. However, when you have something invisible and everything is perfect, I felt like an imposter through the whole thing. I asked, is this really happening?

I was going to many different doctors and I looked at alternative treatments. I called a wonderful clinic in Austria and a place in California and I sent in my biopsies. I wanted to know if there was something else that I could do, did I have to have radiation, and do I have to have chemo? I have estrogen positive HER2 + 3, with a 70% chance of return. Everyone, even some of the alternative clinics, said don't walk to chemo, run. It's a 70% chance to return. When it comes back, it metastasizes, and you will die. This is what they're telling me. However, you don't really understand that. When I read back over my records now, I am appalled. I think I just blanked it out and took it in stride. I decided I just needed to see what I can do. Tt was pretty horrific, as things piled up on each other. I had complications, but I decided that while I was getting the chemo and the radiation, I would also do alternative therapies. I took a very deep dive into high dose vitamin C. The Mayo Clinic, where I was being treated, didn't want me to do ozone therapies, while I was getting the chemo. At one point the cancer moved to my spine, which was a death sentence. They took me off the chemo, because they didn't know what was going on. While I wasn't on chemo, twice a week I got high dose ozone treatments and went into a hyperbaric chamber. Six weeks later, I went back to Mayo. They did another MRI on my spine and another spinal tap. They found that the cancer was gone. It has been two years since my last treatment, and one year since the last surgery. I ended up with a second cancer in my carotid artery.

 Looking back, I think I was in denial. I didn't really believe them. I decided that I would do what they said, because if I didn't, I might die. However, I kept putting off the surgeries and the treatments. I remember I went to Europe first. I was doing crazy stuff and saying that would be back. I became paralyzed one day on the left side of my left arm and leg during a chemo treatment. They thought that maybe I had had a stroke, but this is how they found the enhancement in my spine. When I found out about that, is when it hit home. I think there are two women that lived four years, once the HER2 went into their spine. This is because there is no cure. I was upset and I cried all weekend. This is real, and it is getting real, real fast. This was several months after radiation and the surgeries. This is when I hit it with the ozone treatments. The doctor told me it was gone. I asked the oncologist at Mayo, because I have the MRI's and all the records, where did it go? Do you think the ozone killed it? He just said, I don't know.

During the time when my hair fell out, I lost two of my very dear friends to cancer. Just weeks after my sister shaved the last few hairs on my head, I lost my mother to cancer. It all started hitting home. You think that have this all together, you're doing well, but no not so much. This is when I really fell apart. I had someone significant in my life at that time and it didn't work out. He was wonderful and stayed with me through this. I'm grateful forever for his love and support. I just realized I had to go heal. I had to heal my mind, body and my cells. I knew I had to be better than I was before. I thought I was pretty good before. I thought I was on top of the world. I never questioned why I got the breast cancer diagnosis, I just did. They say we all have cancer cells in us, and sometimes they turn into a full-blown cancer and sometimes they don't.

 I decided that I needed to get it together. I began traveling and went on a spiritual journey. Since I was already into things like ozone therapies and hyperbaric chambers, I went to a place in Costa Rica called

Arrhythmia, where you do Ayahuasca. It is a plant medicine, which is a very healing modality. It heals you from past traumas, current traumas and all kinds of things. While I was there, I met Doctor Mercola. I found out about the biohacking conference. I went to the biohacking conference. I walked in and literally felt like I was at home. These were my people and I wanted all of it. There was cryotherapy, red light therapy and many other therapies. I was running around with a tablet, asking about it all. I just had to have everything. I was going to put it in place, and everybody was going to come and use it. I'm going to help everybody heal!! Then, of course, I started getting the prices on the stuff. I decided to bio hack for three or four months. I stayed in Santa Monica in the Venice Beach area. For four or five days a week I bio hacked. I saw specialists and doctors and continued the journey. Doctor Shallenberger, who's an ozone doctor, tested my mitochondria and found that I was 2% away from osteopenia. I was on hormone blockers. Doctor Shallenberger told me that I have no hormone brain. He wanted to know if I got up and cried every day. I thought I just had chemo brain. Without your hormones, you can't function. Therefore, I decided to go off the hormone blockers. I was supposed to be on them for five years. Mayo kept testing me. They tested my bones and my liver. I asked what they were testing for. They said we're watching as your bones and liver get destroyed, to decide if you need to go off the hormone blocker. Which is the bigger risk, the cancer coming back or the destruction of having no hormones. I didn't like that. Therefore, between my functional naturopathic oncologist in Arizona and Doctor Shallenberger, I went off of the hormone blocker. I decided that I would just test regularly to see what was happening. I started biohacking daily using red light therapy, cryotherapy and pulse electric magnetic field therapy. I also used compression pants, which is a type of lymph drainage system. It also works great for cellulite. I will explain what biohacking is. If you have a hack in the kitchen, such as what is the easiest way to cut a tomato or a papaya. That is a work around or a strategy to make it efficient and optimize your time doing it, so you have the best results. When we bio hack our bodies, we're biohacking our physical body, our mind and our environment. We're using strategies and work arounds to optimize and have the best results possible. It can range from working out, to where you're sleeping, to taking the toxins out of your house. Many of the biohacking modalities, therapies and strategies have been around forever. There are also new scientific things that are crazy cool. You can go off the deep end with it. It works and it is amazing.

After all the biohacking, I had Dr. Shallenberger test my mitochondria. It was an expensive test. However, he turned to me and said that I had the cellular health of a healthy woman in her early 30's. You test mitochondria by testing your rate of exchange of oxygen and how your body is utilizing oxygen. Oxygen is the number one nutrient that our bodies need. Every cell, system, organ and every part of your body needs oxygen to survive and thrive. If you can do this metabolic testing, you can see what your metabolism is doing. How you are using and utilizing oxygen is a direct indication of your cellular health. I also was re-scanned, and my bones are now testing normal with no signs of osteopenia.

I was fortunate that I was able, through this journey, to do ozone treatments. I bought all my own ozone equipment. I have a longevity and ozone sauna at my house. I drink ozone water every day. Ozone is an amazing modality. When you go to a doctor, you can do all of these treatments One of the best things to do is to have your blood ozonated. During my treatment time, when they weren't doing chemo, I went twice a week. I had a port put in that they would take my blood out, mix it with the ozone and process it through an ultraviolet light to also kill viruses and then they put it back in me. After I did that, I would go into a hard-hyperbaric chamber for an hour. You are super hyper oxygenating yourself. When you are under the atmosphere, it's pressing it into your organs and into your circulatory system even more. It clearly gets very expensive. I always knew that I was blessed, because I had the money to do these alternatives. However, it's cost prohibitive for most people. I found that to be very sad. I went out and bought my own equipment. If you can't afford to go to the doctor, they say it's about 90% as effective to do an insufflation rectally, with a bag of ozone. It only costs about a dollar a day, once you make an investment in your own equipment. There are many other things you can do with it. It is great for anti-aging; it puts you in homeostasis and you can use it with acute diseases. It truly is an amazing modality. Part of my journey was that I started collecting this stuff for myself and my mother.

However, I was always very sad about all the people who couldn't afford this. Therefore, my dream is to someday be able to make some sort of place or be able to give back, so that other people can have access to these treatments. I believe that my journey is to share this with people and that growing old is a big fat lie. We do not have to get all bent over and have everything hurt. It's very daunting for people, if you aren't researchers, if they don't read the articles and if they're not into those things. I can just tell you five things to do in the morning, and many people say I can't do that. I think, yes you can because you're doing five things in the morning right now, they are just not the five things I'm doing. What better way to learn than to come stay with me? If you woke up with me and fell asleep with me, I can hold your hand and show you exactly what I do. My dream is to have retreats where participants can experience all the tools firsthand and I can show them how to get the same experiences at home. If I can just get people started and they can see how this can fit into their lifestyle,

this could make a huge impact on their overall energy
and vitality.

Epilogue/Conclusion

I firmly believe that we cannot have true renewed health, until we are ready to get rid of the hidden toxins. For me, that's paying attention to the five pillars of living a toxin free lifestyle; air, water, food, absorption and mental. You see we cannot heal our bodies, if we are not taking our hand away from the fire. Toxins are the fuel feeding the fire that we have to begin removing from our homes and lives. We have toxins everywhere we look. I don't want you to live a life of fear. Just pay attention to what you have control over. That is what is within the four walls of your home. It is said that diet, exercise and environment are the key components contributing to chronic disease. I believe that. Your environment is where you spend your time. It's your office, your home and also the people you are with. The stories I shared with you of mine and others, demonstrated how we have the power to take control of our health. I believe that with every product we use, we are either fighting disease or creating it. The choice is truly yours!

I want to leave you with some resources. First, I have a free toxic risk assessment. The questions will help you look at the potential of risk for you and your family in

all five pillars. It takes less than five minutes to complete. Once you are done, you will get an opportunity to set up a free 10-minute call with me to discuss your results. I can answer any questions you have. I have also created a 5-Day Video course with downloadable resources, guides, and eBooks that will walk you through each room of your house, showing how YOU can create a toxin-free home. You can grab all of this at http:aimeecarlson.com. You'll then get updates from my podcast, The Toxin Terminator, where I share from doctors, experts and industry leaders in the natural health and wellness field and top tips and strategies for living a toxin-free lifestyle. I also hope that you will connect with the community I have on Facebook, The Toxin-Free Lifestyle. I do education and live videos within this community, where I share my best strategies for living a toxin-free lifestyle. You can check out all the toxin-free products I have grown to love and use with my family at:
http://aimeecarlson.com/start

Sources

The Environmental Working Group

The Centers for Disease Control and Prevention

PubMed

The American Cancer Society

The Environmental Protection Agency

The Federal Food and Drug Administration

Safer Cosmetics

Bibliography

(n.d.). Retrieved from Centers for Disease Control and Prevention: https://www.cdc.gov/chronicdisease/index.htm

(n.d.). Retrieved from Medlineplus.gov: https://medlineplus.gov/ency/patientinstructions/000602.htm

(n.d.). Retrieved from EPA: https://www.epa.gov

(n.d.). Retrieved from PubMed: https://www.ncbi.nlm.nih.gov/pmc/articles/PMC3312275/

A Synopsis on Aging-Theories, mechanisms and future prospects. (n.d.). Retrieved from PubMed: https://www.ncbi.nlm.nih.gov/pmc/articles/PMC5991498/

American Cancer Society. (n.d.). Retrieved from cancer.org: https://www.cancer.org/content/dam/cancer-org/research/cancer-facts-and-statistics/annual-cancer-facts-and-figures/2020/cancer-facts-and-figures-2020.pdf

Americans Deserve Better. (n.d.). Retrieved from Non GMO Project: https://www.nongmoproject.org/blog/americans-deserve-better-than-the-usdas-gmo-labeling-law/

Asbestos. (n.d.). Retrieved from Asbestos.com: https://www.asbestos.com/asbestos/statistics-facts/

Authority over Cosmetics. (n.d.). Retrieved from FDA: https://www.fda.gov/cosmetics/cosmetics-laws-regulations/fda-authority-over-cosmetics-how-cosmetics-are-not-fda-approved-are-fda-regulated

Body Effects. (n.d.). Retrieved from American Addiction Centers: https://americanaddictioncenters.org/alcoholism-treatment/body-effects

Breast Cancer & Parabens. (n.d.). Retrieved from WebMD: https://www.webmd.com/breast-cancer/news/20151027/parabens-breast-cancer#1

Class Action Lawsuit. (n.d.). Retrieved from Class Action:
https://www.classaction.com/roundup-weed-killer/lawsuit/

Cosmetic Safety. (n.d.). Retrieved from EWG: https://www.ewg.org/news-
and-analysis/2019/03/cosmetics-safety-us-trails-more-40-nations

Current Health Effects. (n.d.). Retrieved from EMFsinfo:
http://www.emfs.info/health/

Diabetes Data. (n.d.). Retrieved from Centers for Disease Control and
Prevention:
https://www.cdc.gov/diabetes/library/socialmedia/infographics/diabet
es.html

EPA. (n.d.). Retrieved from Advancing Safer Chemicals in Products:
https://www.epa.gov/sites/production/files/2015-09/documents/uml-
rpt_greenpurchasing_7_15_14-2_0.pdf

EWG.ORG. (n.d.). Retrieved from The Environmental Working Group:
https://www.ewg.org/research/minority-cord-blood-report/bpa-and-
other-cord-blood-pollutants

GMO Search. (n.d.). Retrieved from Center For Food Safety:
https://www.centerforfoodsafety.org/search/GMO

Heavy Metals Toxicity and the Environment. (n.d.). Retrieved from PubMed:
https://www.ncbi.nlm.nih.gov/pmc/articles/PMC4144270/

Human Elimination of Phthalates: Blood, Urine & Sweat. (n.d.). Retrieved
from PubMed.org:
https://www.ncbi.nlm.nih.gov/pmc/articles/PMC3504417/

Hunger, poor nutrition lead to chronic disease. (n.d.). Retrieved from Fight
Chronic Disease: https://www.fightchronicdisease.org/latest-
news/hunger-poor-nutrition-lead-chronic-disease

Hyman, D. M. (n.d.). Retrieved from Dr. Hyman:
https://drhyman.com/blog/2010/05/19/is-there-toxic-waste-in-your-
body-2/

*Immunoexcitotoxicity as the central mechanism of etiopathology and
treatment of autism spectrum disorders: A possible role of fluoride*

and aluminum. (n.d.). Retrieved from PubMed:
https://www.ncbi.nlm.nih.gov/pmc/articles/PMC5909100/

Joseph Pizzorno, N. (n.d.). Retrieved from NatureMed:
https://naturemed.org/how-toxins-cause-disease/

Khetan, S. K. (n.d.). *Endocrine Disruptors in the Environment.*

Mental Health. (n.d.). Retrieved from Centers for Disease Control and
Prevention: https://www.cdc.gov/mentalhealth/learn/index.htm

National Children's Study. (n.d.). Retrieved from Centers for Disease Control
and Prevention:
https://www.cdc.gov/biomonitoring/childrens_study.html

National Institute of Health. (n.d.). Retrieved from How Our Body Regulates
Salt Level: https://www.nih.gov/news-events/nih-research-
matters/how-body-regulates-salt-levels

Obesity Rates & Trends Data. (n.d.). Retrieved from State of Childhood
Obesity: https://stateofchildhoodobesity.org/monitor/

Pesticide Use and Exposure Worldwide. (n.d.). Retrieved from PubMed:
https://www.ncbi.nlm.nih.gov/pmc/articles/PMC2946087/

Skin Exposure and Effects. (n.d.). Retrieved from CDC:
https://www.cdc.gov/niosh/topics/skin/default.html

Sleep deprivation and deficiency. (n.d.). Retrieved from National Heart, Lung
and Blood Institute: https://www.nhlbi.nih.gov/health-topics/sleep-
deprivation-and-deficiency

TapWater Database. (n.d.). Retrieved from EWG:
https://www.ewg.org/tapwater/

Wikipedia. (n.d.). Retrieved from
https://en.wikipedia.org/wiki/Bioaccumulation

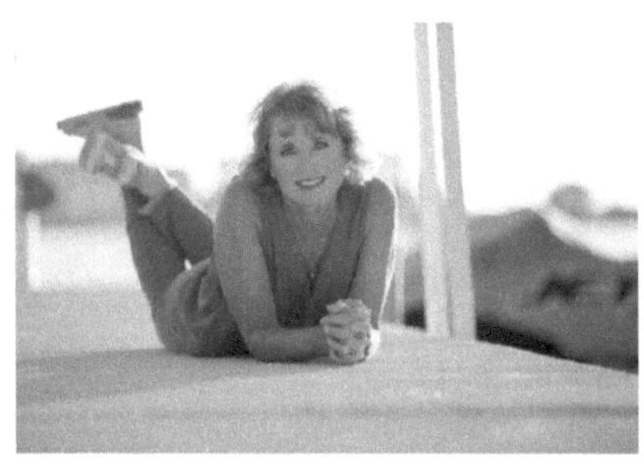

For additional information on Aimee Carlson, go to
www.aimeecarlson.com. To receive updates about author's
books, speaking engagements, events, and more, submit
your info on the subscribe page.

About the Author

Aimee Carlson is a lifetime entrepreneur, having owned and operated a multi-location national franchise, to a professional network marketer, best-selling author and now podcast host of The Toxin Terminator. Aimee is helping people restore and renew their lives, by removing hidden toxins from their homes and their lives. She has spent the last seven years renewing her own health naturally, after working in the automotive industry for many of her adult years. She knew that her toxic exposure was high there. She suffered from migraines, headaches and numerous reproductive problems that led her to have a full hysterectomy at the age of 37 and having to fight menopause symptoms from that time forward. There were many doctor visits, numerous medications, with no solutions. It was truly an accidental opportunity to find solutions that allowed her body to heal. It is now her lifetime purpose and passion to help others find there is a way to live without chronic disease and truly renew their health, focus and energy.